SpringerBriefs in Crin

More information about this series at http://www.springer.com/series/10159

Victoria L. Banyard

Toward the Next Generation of Bystander Prevention of Sexual and Relationship Violence

Action Coils to Engage Communities

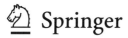

Victoria L. Banyard
Department of Psychology and Prevention
 Innovations Research Center
University of New Hampshire
Durham, NH
USA

ISSN 2192-8533   ISSN 2192-8541   (electronic)
SpringerBriefs in Criminology
ISBN 978-3-319-23170-9   ISBN 978-3-319-23171-6   (eBook)
DOI 10.1007/978-3-319-23171-6

Library of Congress Control Number: 2015947396

Springer Cham Heidelberg New York Dordrecht London
© The Author(s) 2015
This work is subject to copyright. All rights are reserved by the Publisher, whether the whole or part of the material is concerned, specifically the rights of translation, reprinting, reuse of illustrations, recitation, broadcasting, reproduction on microfilms or in any other physical way, and transmission or information storage and retrieval, electronic adaptation, computer software, or by similar or dissimilar methodology now known or hereafter developed.
The use of general descriptive names, registered names, trademarks, service marks, etc. in this publication does not imply, even in the absence of a specific statement, that such names are exempt from the relevant protective laws and regulations and therefore free for general use.
The publisher, the authors and the editors are safe to assume that the advice and information in this book are believed to be true and accurate at the date of publication. Neither the publisher nor the authors or the editors give a warranty, express or implied, with respect to the material contained herein or for any errors or omissions that may have been made.

Printed on acid-free paper

Springer International Publishing AG Switzerland is part of Springer Science+Business Media (www.springer.com)

This book is dedicated to all those who work to support survivors of interpersonal violence as formal and informal helpers and to my father, Richard D. Banyard, who carried forward and modeled a legacy of stepping in to help others

Acknowledgments

Like prevention, this project would not have been possible without the support of many people. In particular, I would like to thank my colleagues at the Prevention Innovations Research Center at the University of New Hampshire, at the New Hampshire Coalition Against Domestic and Sexual Violence, and the National Sexual Violence Resource Center. Their many years of collaboration around prevention and bystander intervention have been the foundation and catalysts for my thinking about this topic. In particular, I thank Mary Moynihan who was my original collaborator in this work and who provided thoughtful edits on earlier drafts of this book. Thank you to my colleagues David Pillemer and Sherry Hamby who planted the idea that I could write a book and encouraged me through the journey. This book is inspired by the dedication of bystander preventionists Bobby Eckstein, Angela Borges, Mary Mayhew, Jane Stapleton, Dorothy Edwards, Alan Berkowitz and many others who have built a legacy of doing change work in communities to promote bystander action. I am also indebted to all the colleagues and students I have had the privilege to work with over the years who keep asking new questions about how we can do prevention better. Most importantly, I wish to thank my family: Dave, Sam, Maggie, and Cameron Howland. Your patience and unwavering support has made possible this project and all of the work leading up to it and from it.

Contents

1	**Introduction**	1
	1.1 Introduction to the Problem	1
	1.2 Aims of the Book	2
	1.3 Defining Terms	3
	1.4 Scope of the Book	3
	References	4
2	**The Promise of a Bystander Approach to Violence Prevention**	7
	2.1 Defining Bystanders	8
	2.2 Defining Prevention	10
	2.3 Defining Sexual and Relationship Violence	10
	2.4 Why Is a Bystander Approach Important?	12
	2.4.1 Bystanders in Primary and Secondary Prevention: The Power of Peer Contexts	12
	2.4.2 Beyond Immediate Relationships: The Role of Bystanders in Community Theories of Violence	14
	2.4.3 Bystanders Are also Part of Tertiary Prevention to Improve Response to Victims and Hold Perpetrators Accountable	16
	2.5 An Introduction to Bystander-Focused Prevention	16
	2.6 Summary	18
	2.7 Implications for Practice	18
	References	19
3	**Pieces of Bystander Action**	25
	3.1 Who	27
	3.1.1 Who Helps?	27
	3.1.2 Who Is Helped?	30
	3.1.3 Perpetrators Versus Victims	30
	3.1.4 Friends Versus Strangers/Ingroup Versus Outgroup	31

	3.2	What or How	32
		3.2.1 Lessons Learned from General Helping and Informal Social Control	32
		3.2.2 Considering the Specifics of SV and IPV	32
	3.3	When	34
		3.3.1 Considering the Type of Situation	34
		3.3.2 Understanding Opportunity to Intervene	36
		3.3.3 Numbers of Other Bystanders	36
		3.3.4 Perceptions of Emergency and Danger	37
		3.3.5 Perceived Barriers to Bystander Action	38
	3.4	Why	39
	3.5	Where	41
		3.5.1 Cultural and Geographic Variability: The Potential Importance of Ecological Niche	41
	3.6	Summary	44
	3.7	Implications for Practice	44
	References		45
4	**Bystander Action Coils: Moving Beyond the Situational Model**		**53**
	4.1	MODELS—Pulling Individual Variables Together	54
	4.2	Limits of Models for Understanding Sexual and Relationship Violence	55
	4.3	Aspects of SV and IPV Bystander Action that Need Attention in a Revised Model	58
		4.3.1 Challenging What Helping Means: The Need for New Scripts	58
		4.3.2 Emphasizing Relational Components of Bystander Action	61
		4.3.3 Embracing a Larger Ecological Model: Revisiting Community and Cultural Factors that Influence Bystander Actions	64
	4.4	Re-envisioning a Model of Bystander Behavior: From Helping Factors to Bystander Action Coils	68
	4.5	Key Points Summary	70
	4.6	Practice Implications	71
	References		72
5	**Building a Better Bystander**		**77**
	5.1	Changing Action Coil 1: Influencing Individual Decision Making	78
		5.1.1 Changing Individual Attitudes	78
		5.1.2 Changing Behavior First	82
		5.1.3 Using Interactions and Relationships to Change Attitudes	84

		5.1.4	Addressing More Than One Attitude at a Time	86
		5.1.5	Accounting for Individual Differences in Attitude Change Approaches	87
	5.2	Changing Action Coil 2: Contextual Processes		88
		5.2.1	Change Community Leaders and Engage Early Adopters	88
		5.2.2	Changing Norms	89
		5.2.3	Policy Change Can Impact Individual Action	94
	5.3	Changing Action Coil 3: Influencing the Event Itself		96
		5.3.1	Social Scripts	96
	5.4	Changing Action Coil 4: Influencing Outcomes		97
		5.4.1	Action Effectiveness	98
		5.4.2	Building Collective Efficacy	99
		5.4.3	Training Professional Responders	100
		5.4.4	Bystanders Supporting Bystanders	100
		5.4.5	Safety Nets for Bystanders	101
	5.5	Summary		101
	5.6	Practice Implications		102
	References			103
6	**Prevention Springs from Action Coils: A Strategic Plan for Comprehensive Bystander-Focused Prevention**			**111**
	6.1	General Principles of Next Generation Bystander Prevention Approaches		112
		6.1.1	Comprehensive Mobilization	112
		6.1.2	Building New Helping Scripts	113
		6.1.3	Expanding View of Bystander Roles	113
		6.1.4	Consequences of Bystander Action	114
	6.2	Prevention Across Levels and Settings of the Ecological Model		114
	6.3	Promoting Bystander Action Across the Lifespan: Developmental Leverage Points		116
	6.4	Conclusion		117
	References			117

Chapter 1
Introduction

> *It's hard to help if it's like a group of people and no one else is doing anything, it's easy to just fall into the crowd and not do anything.*
> —College student discussing helping related to sexual and relationship violence

Abstract The epidemic of sexual and relationship violence in communities is well documented. While *interventions* to assist victims have proliferated in the last several decades, *prevention* of this problem remains understudied. Bystander intervention is a promising prevention innovation that gives everyone a role to play in ending violence by promoting collective efficacy and a sense of responsibility combined with skills for stepping into help others and to change social norms. This chapter describes the aims of the book and the scope of what will be covered.

Keywords Bystander · Sexual violence · Relationship abuse

1.1 Introduction to the Problem

The epidemic of sexual and relationship violence in communities is well documented. The recent National Sexual Violence and Intimate Partner Violence Survey estimated that one in five women experience rape in their lifetime (45 % report some other type of unwanted sexual experience) and men also report both of these types of victimization. Nearly one third of women in the NISVS sample reported experiencing physical violence by an intimate partner (Black et al. 2011). While *interventions* to assist victims have proliferated in the last several decades, *prevention* of this problem remains understudied. The need to improve our efforts is clear as we tally the numbers of victims and the toll of negative physical and mental health consequences they experience as a result of sexual and relationship violence (Black et al. 2011). We know that sexual and relationship violence are not just individual problems. While a perpetrator's behavior is linked to his own exposure to violence and ways of thinking that see sexual intimacy as adversarial, it is also promoted by the community—by friends who support the use of coercion in relationships, bartenders or teachers who look the other way when demeaning comments are made or when someone's personal boundaries are encroached upon, neighbors who lack a sense of trust and common purpose with one another, and social policies that do not adequately address social disorganization (Lippy and DeGue 2015; Tharp et al. 2012). Thus our prevention efforts should be broader than potential perpetrators or victims (Banyard et al. 2003; DeGue et al. 2014). Bystander intervention is a promising prevention innovation (Katz 1995). It gives everyone a role to play in ending violence by promoting collective efficacy and a sense of responsibility combined with skills for stepping into help others and to change social norms.

1.2 Aims of the Book

Bystander intervention has been explored in research studies across many disciplines and implemented by practitioners. Yet to date, there has been little synthesis of this research and bridging between it and the practices of advocates and preventionists. What is more, the model of bystander intervention on which current prevention programs are based is not up to the task of describing the many forces that hinder and promote taking action in situations of sexual and relationship violence. The purpose of this book is to integrate research about who helps others and under what conditions, including when there is risk for victimization. I present a revised model to explain bystander responses. With this knowledge in hand, communities can develop a prevention agenda that more effectively calls bystanders to action, empowering these critical players to reduce sexual and partner violence.

Along the way, the book will address the following questions: What is the promise of a bystander approach to violence prevention? Where does it fit within the spectrum of sexual and relationship violence prevention? How do we expand theoretical models of helping behavior to the unique context of interpersonal violence? How can we bring in research from other areas of health behavior change and developmental research on violence to inform a broader bystander intervention model? What practices might follow from a revised model of bystander action? Research and practices related to bystanders and sexual and relationship violence prevention have mainly involved college students and that will form the basis for the work reviewed here. However, the purpose of the book is to develop a model that is also informed by community-based work and school-based work with younger students. The aim is to produce an expanded model of bystander intervention on which a next generation of bystander prevention strategies can be built.

1.3 Defining Terms

But what is a bystander? Bystanders are individuals or groups of individuals who are present when someone needs help or when some sort of negative behavior (like bullying or harassing comments) is taking place. They are not themselves in need of help or instigators of the problem and thus have the potential to make the situation better. Activities in which bystanders might engage include directly providing assistance to someone at risk of victimization, confronting a potential perpetrator, enlisting friends of a victims to intervene, saying something or calling in professional helpers like police (e.g. McMahon and Banyard 2012 for a review related to sexual violence). Building future bystander prevention practices must be grounded in lessons learned from theories and empirical studies of bystander action across settings. Perhaps the most obvious role for bystanders is in helping the person who needs help (the victim in the case of crimes). This has been the focus of most social psychological theories and research on bystander behavior as well as on helping and altruism more generally (Penner et al. 2005). Sociological theories of informal social control have added to the literature describing how bystanders get involved in addressing perpetrators or individuals who engage in rule- or norm-violating behavior. Because violence prevention is also related to social justice issues (Katz et al. 2011), research related to engaging individuals in activities to promote more sustained engagement in ending violence through community education, resource building, policy changes should also be considered.

1.4 Scope of the Book

Chapter 2 provides an overview of why bystanders are important for the prevention of sexual and intimate partner violence. I then review in Chap. 3 how bystander behaviors, and helpful bystander actions in particular, happen. What factors have been studied and what key models help us understand who acts, when and why? I use the ecological model to summarize variables within the individual, within relationships, proximal situational factors as well as broader social context norms and policies that have been found relevant to understanding bystander action. This chapter also highlights limitations of current conceptualizations of bystander behavior. Chapter 4 describes an expanded model for understanding bystander action. This model incorporates lessons learned from empirical research on bystander behavior across many different disciplines and topics to describe a more comprehensive framework of bystander action in the unique and challenging context of sexual and relationship violence. While much of the work on which this new model is based was conducted on college campuses with young adults, the model is also informed by community based research and investigations of younger students in middle and high school. Prevention seeks not only to understand bystanders but to get them to change their attitudes, and ultimately their behaviors so that they are more motivated to step in and better able to be helpful in ways that are skilled and protect their own safety in risky situations. They are also potential diffusers of innovations (Cook-Craig et al. 2014; Rogers 2002), individuals who can role model new community norms to change broader cultural stories that support violence. Further, bystanders are potential gatekeepers to policy and resource changes (as college administrators or faculty, school principals, community and spiritual leaders) at the community level, individuals who with a changed perspective may have the power and influence to better support services for victims, community responses to perpetrators and more proactive prevention efforts.

Thus, in Chap. 5 I explore what we know about behavior change, including links between changing attitudes and beliefs and actually impacting behavior. Applications to prevention of sexual and relationship violence are noted throughout the book, particularly in brief practice implication sections at the end of each chapter. However, in the final chapter I tie all of these threads together, outlining a strategic plan for bystander focused prevention that moves beyond limitations of current models. This chapter considers the place of bystander intervention in comprehensive, multi-pronged approaches to violence prevention, describes new key components that should be included in bystander intervention based on the integrated model presented in Chap. 4, and highlights how such a prevention plan can be flexible so that it really works in a variety of individual communities. Throughout the book I use quotes from young adults reflecting on bystander experiences from studies of rural communities and a college campus. (Banyard et al. 2014; Edwards et al. 2014). College campuses are the most studied but are only one location for bystander intervention, and this book draws from research in community as well as secondary school settings. However, college campuses are the locations most widely studied and thus provide many of the most accessible examples of constructs.

References

Banyard, V., Moynihan, M. M., Wible, E., & Johnson, M. (2014). *Reflections on bystander intervention: College students discuss sexual violence and relationship abuse prevention*. Manuscript in preparation.

Banyard, V. L., Plante, E. G., & Moynihan, M. M. (2003). Bystander education: Bringing a broader community perspective to sexual violence prevention. *Journal of Community Psychology, 32*, 61–79.

Black, M.C., Basile, K.C., Breiding, M.J., Smith, S.G., Walters, M.L., & Merrick, M.T., et al. (2011). The National Intimate Partner and Sexual Violence Survey (NISVS): 2010 Summary Report. Atlanta, GA: National Center for Injury Prevention and Control, Centers for Disease Control and Prevention.

Cook-Craig, P. G., Coker, A. L., Clear, E. R., Garcia, L. S., Bush, H. M., Brancato, C. J., et al. (2014). Challenge and opportunity in evaluating a diffusion-based active bystanding prevention program green dot in high schools. *Violence Against Women, 20*, 1179–1202.

DeGue, S., Valle, A., Holt, M. K., Massetti, G. M., Matjasko, J. L., & Tharp, A. T. (2014). A systematic review of primary prevention strategies for sexual violence perpetration. *Aggression and Violent Behavior, 19*, 346–362.

References

Edwards, K., Mattingly, M. J., Dixon. K. J., & Banyard, V. L. (2014). Community matters: Intimate partner violence among young adults. *American Journal of Community Psychology, 53*, 198–207.

Katz, J. (1995). Reconstructing masculinity in the locker room: The mentors in violence prevention project. *Harvard Educational Review, 65*, 163–174.

Katz, J., Heisterkamp, A., & Flemming, A. M. (2011). The social justice roots of the mentors in violence prevention model and its application to a high school setting. *Violence Against Women, 17*, 684–702.

Lippy, C., & DeGue, S. (2015). Exploring alcohol policy approaches to prevent sexual violence perpetration. *Trauma, Violence, & Abuse.*

McMahon, S., & Banyard, V. L. (2012). When can I help? A conceptual framework for the prevention of sexual violence through bystander intervention. *Trauma, Violence, & Abuse, 13*, 3–14.

Penner, L. A., Dovidio, J. F., Piliavin, J. A., & Schroeder, D. A. (2005). Prosocial behavior: Multilevel perspectives. *Annual Review of Psychology, 56*, 365–392.

Rogers, E. M. (2002). Diffusion of preventive innovations. *Addictive Behaviors, 27*, 989–993.

Tharp, A. T., DeGue, S., Valle, L. A., Brookmeyer, K. A., Massetti, G. M., & Matjasko, J. L. (2012). A systematic qualitative review of risk and protective factors for sexual violence perpetration. *Trauma, Violence, & Abuse, 14*, 133–167.

Chapter 2
The Promise of a Bystander Approach to Violence Prevention

> *Some of my friends in the dorm were like 'why would you-why would you even get involved like it's none of your business it's better for you to just stay uninvolved' And I think that's just weird because that's just not the type of person I am.*
> —College student discussing being a bystander

Abstract Bystander intervention has provided a new way to approach sexual and relationship violence prevention. It gives everyone a role to play in prevention that is appealing and that potentially reduces defensiveness to prevention messages. This chapter provides an introduction to bystander focused prevention for sexual and relationship violence. Definitions of key terms including bystanders, prevention, and violence concepts are provided. Support for the importance of bystanders to the topic of sexual and relationship abuse comes from a variety of theories about the causes of sexual and relationship violence and research on risk and protective factors. Theories and research across all levels of the social ecological model are briefly reviewed to make the case for the utility of using a bystander approach to violence prevention.

Keywords Sexual assault · Relationship violence · Bystanders · Theory

Sexual and relationship violence prevention efforts have been around for many years. Yet programs often show limited success. Even if, for example, individuals profess to endorse fewer rape myths immediately after sitting through a rape prevention workshop, these shifts often disappear weeks and months later. Few programs examine their effect on rates of sexual or relationship violence. Researchers and practitioners have critiqued early prevention approaches for talking to women mainly as potential victims and to men as potential perpetrators. Not surprisingly, such frameworks produced resistance to messages and engagement (Lonsway 1996; Lonsway et al. 2009). Other programs focused less on prevention for women and more on risk reduction training (Gidycz and Dardis 2014). Bystander intervention gives *everyone* a positive role to play in violence prevention.

Further, prevention work often consists of presentations focused on building knowledge and awareness among those individuals most at risk (for example, college students) (Anderson and Whiston 2005; DeGue et al. 2014). In order for prevention to be effective, approaches that get people more personally connected to the material and approaches that find ways to engage many components of community (for example, parents as well as students), and that have concrete skill building to offer will be more effective at helping people do something different to end sexual and relationship violence (Finkehor et al. 2014; DeGue et al. 2012). Bystander intervention is more appealing and potentially reduces defensiveness to prevention messages. While it may be hard for a high school student to see herself as a potential victim of relationship abuse and a staff member at a youth based organization to see himself as a potential perpetrator of sexual violence, both of them are likely eager to have the skills to help a friend or family member who is dealing with abuse or to know how to safely de-escalate a risky situation where someone is in danger of being hurt. Further, changing community norms, implementing better policies, and resourcing comprehensive prevention efforts that will work, relies on communities of leaders and citizens who are aware of the problems of SV and IPV, feel responsible for doing something about it, and take action. As a potential added benefit, as bystanders learn how to help others they may also adopt new ways of thinking and acting that may reduce their own victimization or perpetration risk. Thus the prevention field has turned to trying to motivate and create better bystanders.

2.1 Defining Bystanders

Bystanders have been defined in many different ways in both research and practice. Most definitions describe bystanders as witnesses to negative behavior (an emergency, a crime, rule violating behavior) who by their presence have the opportunity to step into provide help, contribute to the negative behavior or encourage it in some way, or stand by and do nothing but observe. Bystanders who do take action have been referred to in the literature as "upstanders" (Ferrans et al. 2012; Twemlow and Sacco 2013), "defenders" (Pozzoli et al. 2012), active or empowered bystanders or pro-social bystanders (Banyard 2011) to help distinguish them from people who "stand-by" and do nothing in these situations or those who may escalate the problem.

Historically some of the earliest research on bystanders examined their apathy, or lack of action. Darley and Latané (1968) used the term "diffusion of responsibility" to describe why bystanders in large groups in particular, are less likely to help in part because they assume others will take care of the situation. In Richmond California in October of 2009 (CNN, 28 October, 2009) and again in Steubenville, Ohio in 2012 young women were incapacitated by alcohol and gang raped while school peers watched, texted their friends, and videotaped events (Dahl 2013). No one stepped into help either young woman. In a high school in Massachusetts in 2013 a young man was sexually assaulted as part of a hazing incident while others looked on (Adams 2013). On one college campus, a victim of stalking came forward to both campus authorities and law enforcement. Friends of the perpetrator then flooded Facebook with negative and harassing comments about her. In this case the bystanders mobilized to make the situation worse by blaming the victim and disparaging her for coming forward. The recent trial of two students at Vanderbilt University described a sexual assault where a number of people witnessed the victimization and did nothing including friends of the perpetrators who received videos and texts about the assault (Burke 2015). In New Jersey, several college students were recently arrested for their roles as bystanders who assisted several accused perpetrators in a sexual assault (Cohen 2014).

On the other hand, social psychological work on altruism and helping as well as more contemporary work on bystanders has examined when people step into assist others (Penner et al. 2005). At the University of Massachusetts several students came to the aid of a young woman during an assault and assisted the campus with identifying the perpetrator (Winerip 2014). In Steubenville, Ohio, an online blogger refused to be silent about what she read and heard online about the sexual assault of a high school student (Preston 2013). At Stanford University two students riding their bikes intervened to stop a man who was having sex with a young woman who appeared unconscious (Lee 2015). At Vanderbilt University officials were looking at surveillance cameras related to a different situation and noticed a young woman being taken unconscious by the accused men to their room. Hightened sensitivity to the context of sexual assault risk and what it looks like helped these more formally trained bystanders attend to this section of footage and they initiated an investigation that resulted in two men being convicted of sexual assault related crimes (Gonzalez 2015). In this book, I mainly focus on this latter group, individuals who choose to take action in situations across the spectrum of sexual and relationship violence.

Research using national crime data found that a third party was present in one third of sexual assaults and one third of instances of intimate partner violence, according to victim reports (Planty 2002). Victims most often said that third parties made the situation better (Planty 2002). Bystanders are also present across a variety of interpersonal violence situations (including peer bullying, child maltreatment, intimate partner violence, and sexual assault) (Hamby et al. 2015). Bystanders were least likely to be present for sexual assaults, but when bystanders were present they were often helpful, though they also were at risk of being hurt. Many incoming college students performed a prosocial bystander action related to sexual assault in the past year (McMahon et al. 2015). High numbers of students reported that they had opportunity to do these behaviors and that when presented with the opportunity most did something to try to help. These data suggest that informal helpers are often present and can offer help. Bystanders are, however, frequently unsure of themselves as responders. They are unclear about whether intervention is needed or welcomed or what they should do to help (Break the Cycle, 2006; Knowledge Networks 2011).

2.2 Defining Prevention

Prevention of violence can take place at each of three levels of prevention (Centers for Disease Control Prevention 2004; O'Connell et al. 2009): primary, secondary, or tertiary. Primary prevention involves efforts aimed universally at an entire population and usually aim to keep the problem from developing in the first place. Secondary prevention involves more targeted efforts. An at-risk group is identified and efforts are put in place to reduce those risk factors to keep the problem from developing further. Tertiary prevention can also be seen as intervention in that it takes place after violence has taken place. The goal is to work with victims to reduce the negative consequences and decrease experiencing future victimization or to work with perpetrators to rehabilitate and reduce recidivism. Bystanders can play a role in each of these types of prevention.

2.3 Defining Sexual and Relationship Violence

Bystanders have the opportunity to respond to a wide array of situations related to sexual (SV) and intimate partner or relationship violence (IPV). For the purposes of the current discussion and consistent with the field I use a variety of terms when referring to SV (sexual assault, sexual violence) and IPV (dating violence, relationship abuse) and include a range of behaviors in each category. For example, bystanders can take action across a range of behaviors that can indicate risk for sexual violence including sexist comments and verbal harassment (e.g. catcalls); comments that minimize rape (e.g. "that test raped me"); unwanted touching and groping; engaging in sexual behavior with someone who is too incapacitated to give consent; sexual assault using force or threats of force (McMahon and Banyard 2012). A similar continuum can be described for relationship abuse with behaviors ranging from inappropriate comments that depict physical abuse in relationships humorously, comments that suggest support for coercion in relationships, warning signs of abuse including jealous and controlling behavior, insulting or demeaning one's partner, stalking, and acts of physical abuse or threats of physical abuse. A continuum approach is similar to the "Broken Windows" or social disorganization theory of crime (Perkins et al. 1992; Pinchevesky and Wright 2012; Wilson and Kelling 1982). The idea is that small acts of social disorganization such as broken windows on a building or sexist or misogynist comments suggest social and community norms in favor of negative behaviors, and these small actions and attitudes breed the norms that condone larger and larger problems. Appreciating the spectrum of these behaviors is an important context for understanding the variety of unique opportunities and challenges for bystanders to sexual and relationship violence, the main subject of this book.

In this book I take an interconnected view of violence given the high rates of co-occurrence of different forms of violence (Hamby and Grych 2013). Meaningful prevention efforts across the lifespan should consider more than one type of violence as a focus for any given effort especially since while distinct types of violence have some specific risk and protective factors, they also have many in common (Hamby and Grych 2013). Risk factors such as bystander apathy and lack of collective efficacy, community and peer norms that support the use of violence and coercion, are related to many forms of violence and could be a common focus for prevention work. We know from research that individuals have difficulties identifying escalating risk for both SV and IPV and that privacy norms support seeing both forms of interpersonal violence as a personal and private matter. We know both forms of violence occur on a continuum ranging from comments, jokes, harassment and emotional abuse to problematic physical contact and both often occur behind closed doors. Further, while most research has focused on bystanders in relation to only one form of interpersonal violence per study, making direct comparisons difficult, factors related to bystander action often appear similar. Thus in the current book I often describe a bystander approach to interpersonal violence more generally.

However, when possible I also explore how bystander intervention may be somewhat different depending on whether it is in relation to sexual violence or relationship abuse, or other forms of interpersonal violence. For example, one study found that bystanders were less likely to be present for sexual assaults and when they were, bystanders were more likely to have been reported as harmed than for other forms of victimization (Hamby et al. 2015). Sexual assaults also frequently occur when victims have been given alcohol or substances that incapacitate them and make it difficult for them to provide cues that help is needed or that they would be receptive to bystander intervention (I should note that it is not the responsibility of victims to indicate their need for help—the responsibility for sexual assault rests with perpetrators—but absent verbal or non-verbal communication with victims, bystanders who are feeling unsure about taking action may be more likely to walk away from the situation). Norms about how sexual interactions happen also work against bystanders identifying instances of risk for sexual assault. Sexual scripts that encourage men to be persistent in pursuing sexual contact or that support ideas that "no means yes," that encourage gender segregated socializing, and that pair aggression with sexuality pervade media images and may desensitize or confuse bystanders about cues that risk for SV may be escalating (Abbey et al. 2001; McCauley et al. 2012; Menning 2009), though some studies find high levels of intervention by bystanders in sexual assault situations (Harari et al. 1985).

IPV also has unique aspects for bystanders (Frye et al. 2012). Threatening physical postures and emotionally abusive name calling and insults may in some instances be more recognizable as a problem in the eyes of a bystander and studies find reports of high levels of responding to IPV with responses like providing advice or support or admonishing the perpetrator, especially compared to reporting to police (Gracia et al. 2009). Yet norms of privacy may hinder taking action. In the case of IPV, bystanders may be concerned for their own safety more than with other forms of interpersonal violence, if they step in when someone is being physically violent. More lab based studies showed that gender of the perpetrator was key, with earlier work suggesting people were less likely to intervene if they thought the people involved were a couple (Shotland and Straw 1976), and more recent work suggests that people are more likely to take action in an IPV situation if the perpetrator is male (Chabot et al. 2009). A more community-based study found that individuals thought the most feasible forms of bystander action related to IPV were trying to help a victim (Frye et al. 2012). By contrast, college students were most likely to report having intervened as bystanders to sexual violence in escalating risk situations by trying to reduce or diffuse the risk (McMahon et al. 2015).

To date, few studies have sought to examine differences in bystander action for SV and IPV by comparing them directly. Some research that has, for example, compared correlates of helping for general violence compared to IPV found some different correlates (taking action against general violence was more likely among those with strong social support ties to neighbors while action for IPV was related to less personal tolerance of IPV) but also similarities (self-efficacy was significantly related to informal social control of both) (Frye 2007). As a result, in this book I attempt to create a broad model that is applicable to mobilizing bystanders for SV and IPV but also note the need for future research to examine more unique aspects of SV and IPV for bystanders that should be further developed.

2.4 Why Is a Bystander Approach Important?

Support for the importance of bystanders to the topic of sexual and relationship abuse comes from a variety of theories about the causes of sexual and relationship violence and research on risk and protective factors. Variables focus on aspects of individuals, relationship contexts, and communities (Tharp et al. 2012; Vagi and Rothman 2013). Indeed, it is possible to find an important role for bystanders in many of the most supported theories of sexual violence and relationship abuse. A brief review of this work sets an important context for understanding the potential of bystanders for prevention across levels of the social ecological model (Tharp et al. 2012; Vagi and Rothman 2013). Bystanders have the greatest potential for changing the environment and relationships that surround potential perpetrators.

2.4.1 Bystanders in Primary and Secondary Prevention: The Power of Peer Contexts

The most well studied and supported risk factors for perpetration of SV and IPV are found at the intra-individual level of the social ecology (Tharp et al. 2012; Vagi and Rothman 2013 for reviews). Risk factors such as patterns of thinking including belief in rape myths, victim blaming attitudes, as well as a history of victimization or witnessing violence, and patterns of sexual behavior including impersonal sex and sexual arousal to aggressive stimuli (Capaldi et al. 2012; Tharp et al. 2012). There may be little influence that bystander intervention can have on internal patterns of thought, sexual arousal, and motivation to use coercion and aggression in relationships in the moment someone is making the choice to hurt another. However, we know that intra-individual factors do not operate in isolation. For example, several theories of perpetration highlight how individual risk factors are combined with contextual factors to produce perpetration behaviors (Tharp et al. 2012). Bystanders play a role in increasing or decreasing these additional contextual factors. For example, qualitative interviews with men who self reported behaviors that would meet legal definitions of rape and yet did not see what they had done as wrong or criminal found in the men's description of the rapes many bystanders who helped, knowingly or not, create the context that made it easy for these men to perpetrate their crimes (Lisak and Miller 2001). Bystanders were the friends and acquaintances who helped set up the party, made alcohol available, set up rooms where one could isolate a victim, and looked the other way when risk began to escalate. Indeed, on college campuses researchers observed different social interaction patterns in fraternities students described as high risk compared to those perceived as lower risk for sexual assault. High risk fraternity parties showed greater gender segregation at social events, use of aggression more generally in social interactions, and conversations between men and women characterized by more straight flirting rather than friendly general conversations (Boswell and Spade 1996; Humphrey and Kahn 2000; Menning 2009).

With regard to IPV, bystanders are the neighbors in communities beyond college campuses who by not seeing IPV as a problem may look the other way and thus allow abuse in relationships to take place (Frye 2007; Rothman et al. 2011a, b). Routine activities theory (Schwartz et al. 2001) specifies that three key variables are necessary for a crime to occur: The presence of a motivated perpetrator, a vulnerable potential victim, and the absence of "effective guardians" who could take action. These guardians are bystanders and have the potential to interrupt and prevent crime an individual chooses to commit. For example, research on bullying is clear that bystanders who step up and defend bullied children reduce rates of bullying in schools while bullies who are rewarded or reinforced for their behaviors escalate the problem (Salmivalli et al. 2011). Bystanders, then, can work against a perpetrator's choice to use violence in a relationship. Bystanders in these models are key factors in primary and universal prevention efforts in that they may keep violence from happening in the first place.

Beyond simply interrupting behaviors, bystanders are also part of the immediate context of SV and IPV as part of the peer norms that can support or work against SV and IPV, the relationship level of the social ecological model. Again, research on perpetration of both SV and IPV shows that peer pressure for sexual activity, peer support for forced sex, membership in hypermasculine peer groups are risk factors for perpetration (Tharp et al. 2012). Social norms theory describes how problematic behaviors are encouraged because of misperceptions of how much peers engage or support those behaviors (Paul and Gray 2011). So, while men may not hold rape myths themselves, they may overestimate how much their peers endorse rape myths and over time bring their own behavior in line with perceived peer expectations (Fabiano et al. 2003). Further, men who do not seek and receive consent before sexual behavior may think their behavior is normative. The solution to these misperceptions is to provide corrective norm information. This can come in part from prevention messages (Fabiano et al. 2003) but also needs to come from peer bystanders who challenge these misperceptions in conversation and in modelling different behaviors. Among high school students, more gender equitable attitudes were associated with lower risk for perpetrating dating violence. Witnessing peers perpetrate abuse increased risk for perpetration among research participants (McCauley et al. 2013). Bystanders are part of these peer groups and may work to support or challenge these norms as well as model positive or negative behavior that can be part of cultural tipping points for encouraging violence or preventing it. In this way they are also a key component of secondary prevention as they counteract the problematic views that make some individuals more likely to perpetrate.

2.4.2 Beyond Immediate Relationships: The Role of Bystanders in Community Theories of Violence

Social disorganization theory (Lippy and DeGue 2014; Pinchevsky and Wright 2012) is also relevant to understanding the potential role of bystanders. This theory describes how neighborhood factors, including economic resources, neighborhood disorganization, as well as relationships between members of the community impact the occurrence of crime (Edwards et al. 2014; Frye et al. 2012; Malik et al. 1997; Rothman et al. 2011a, b; Snyder et al. 2012; Weiss 2011). The idea of this is that things like high rates of poverty and the stress and disadvantage that can accompany it leave people in communities with few resources to form ties and little power to work together on common goals. There is then a dearth of cooperation to reduce crime and individuals may be less willing to use their own influence to keep risky situations from escalating (termed informal social control (Chaurand and Brauer 2008; Chekroun and Brauer 2002). In situations of high social capital and collective efficacy, people use the relationships they have with one another to exert control over the behavior of others but also to create norms and rules that can promote collaborative action and achieving common goals. There is evidence that third parties are less likely to be involved in crimes in urban areas, where perhaps due to social disorganization there is less community cohesion, compared to rural or suburban towns (Planty 2002).

Indeed, researchers have found that measures of collective efficacy were correlated with violence. That is, communities high in collective efficacy had members who looked out for one another and were able to work together on crime prevention efforts, neighborhood youth monitoring, and promoting prosocial community norms. They had social bonds and ties that enabled neighbors or groups of people to work collaboratively together, to forms shared goals and then help achieve them. Young adults who felt they were part of rural communities with

2.4 Why Is a Bystander Approach Important?

greater collective efficacy also reported that they took more bystander action, while neighborhoods seen by citizens as unorganized and lacking cohesion had high rates of relationship violence (Edwards et al. 2014; Rothman et al. 2011a, b), though work in urban studies has not found a significant link between collective efficacy and IPV intervention or rates of femicide (Frye et al. 2007, 2008). Women who felt more positively about their communities also reported social norms that were more supportive of helping women in abusive relationships (McDonnell et al. 2011). Social capital has been used as a resource to reduce adolescent crime (Weiss 2011).

Building relationships within communities are then a key part of building protective factors against violence. Bystanders are the broad base of human and social capital needed to bring about change. In this way they serve the efforts of secondary prevention, by being more present at "hot spots" where SV and IPV are more likely to occur (Taylor et al. 2013), or by intervening as part of collective groups as violence escalates to promote nonviolent outcomes (Levine et al. 2011).

Bystanders are also potential community change agents in more direct ways than through their role in helping to create community norms, capital and collective efficacy. "Diffusion of Innovation theory" describes the process through which new ideas and actions (for example, new ideas about relationships, violence, or prevention) spread among people so that they take root in a community (Rogers 2002). The process of diffusion enlists small groups of "innovators" and "early adopters" who are often people others look up to as opinion leaders in a group or community (Rogers 2002). When they see the relative advantage of the new idea or action they can encourage others so that the new norms or actions become more widespread. Bystanders have a role as these potential innovators or early adopters of violence prevention messages and behavior choices. However, bystanders act in such roles (by, for example, seeking out information about SV or IPV and educating others) infrequently (McMahon et al. 2015).

Frye et al. (2012) found that neighborhood residents generated a number of ways that community engagement could be used to address IPV, by getting leaders to speak out against IPV and working to create safe community spaces. Citizens also thought these sorts of strategies were somewhat to very effective, though lower rated than directly trying to help a victim or contacting a formal helping system. Bystanders can be gatekeepers of community-level change. Policy contexts also impact SV and IPV (Lippy and DeGue 2014; Taylor et al. 2013). Community leaders and people in power are the gatekeepers of policy changes. They have authority to resource supports for victims, provide training for better response to perpetrators, and policies that indicate zero tolerance for coercion. For example, researchers have discussed "decision and deterrence theories" (Paul and Gray 2011, p. 105) which highlight the need for real negative consequences for negative behaviors like IPV or SV as perceived consequences can make a difference in whether a perpetrator chooses to act (Strang and Peterson 2013). Bystanders can lobby for creation of and enforcement of consequences for problems like SV and IPV. This can be seen, for example, in the recent work of student activists who have pressured college campus leaders to make changes in how instances of sexual assault are handled on campus.

2.4.3 Bystanders Are also Part of Tertiary Prevention to Improve Response to Victims and Hold Perpetrators Accountable

The importance of focusing on bystanders is also supported by research on what happens to victims after they experience a sexual assault or relationship abuse. At that point in time bystanders are the friends, family members, and first responders who hear victims talk about their experiences and can offer support and referral to resources or provide negative responses that silence victims and compound their distress. For example, we know from studies that victims often receive both helpful and unhelpful reactions from others when they talk about their victimization (West and Wandrei 2002; Ullman 2010). Supportive reactions from others predicted recovery from sexual assault and relationship abuse while negative reactions were associated with psychological distress (Ullman 2010). Victim blaming attitudes from professional helpers can also be damaging (Campbell 1998, 2001). Furthermore, from a victims' perspective, bystanders are associated with more positive victim mental health and fewer negative effects following the victimization, though it is not just the presence of bystanders, the bystanders have to be perceived as helpful and victims need to perceive that bystanders are safe and not harmed in the situation (Hamby et al. 2015). Bystanders, then, also play an important role in tertiary prevention, in reducing further effects of violence by being a key part of safety nets for victims in the aftermath of sexual violence or relationship abuse.

It is also the case that bystanders can become witnesses not only by alerting law enforcement when a crime has occurred but by providing evidence for investigations and testimony in legal cases or campus judicial board hearings. One study found arrest rates were significantly increased for IPV in a community when bystanders gave sworn testimony or became complainants themselves (Buzawa and Austin 1993; Shernock 2005).

2.5 An Introduction to Bystander-Focused Prevention

From these theories and frustration at the lack of effectiveness of prior prevention efforts, prevention educators developed programs aimed at changing the attitudes and building the capacity of potential bystanders. A central theme in bystander focused prevention is that everyone has a role to play in ending sexual and relationship violence. In their role as friends, family, neighbors, co-workers, or strangers in a bar or on the street, they may notice situations of escalating risk for violence or become aware of the abuse of power in relationships. They have the opportunity before, during, and also after an incident to find ways to help. Harnessing this potential is the focus of many prevention programs. These programs provide more evidence for the importance of attending to bystanders as several studies suggest that these prevention programs may help prevent violence (Coker et al. 2014; Salazar et al. 2014).

Katz's Mentors in Violence Prevention (MVP) (Katz 1995) and Berkowitz's (Gidycz et al. 2011) Men's Project are two of the founding programs on bystander intervention for sexual and relationship violence. They focus on small group, single gender workshops that raise awareness about the problem but also use active learning exercises such as reviewing and role playing scenarios and challenging social norms through discussion to increase helpful bystander behaviors. Since their early work many other programs have appeared using similar educational workshop formats (Bringing in the Bystander™ (Banyard et al. 2007), Men of Strength Clubs (Men Can Stop Rape), GreenDot and SEEDS (Coker et al. 2011, 2014; Cook-Craig 2014), One in Four Men's and Women's Program (Foubert and Newberry 2006). A bystander framework has also been used to develop other types of prevention tools including social marketing campaigns (Know Your Power™, Red Flag Campaign), interactive theatre (iSCREAM, interACT) and online curricula (PETSA at the University of Montana, RealConsent at Emory, and Agent of Change We End Violence, Take Care) and some of these have been evaluated with promising results (Ahrens et al. 2011; Kleinsasser et al. 2015 ; McMahon et al. 2014; Potter 2012; Salazar et al. 2014). Katz and Moore's (2013) recent meta-analysis shows the promise of this approach.

In this book I take a closer look at this new tool in our prevention toolkit—mobilizing potential bystanders to play a role in ending violence. A bystander framework is one facet of interpersonal violence prevention. Empirical research supports attention to risk reduction, for example (Gidycz and Dardis 2014), parent education (i.e., dyadic intervention for parents of entering college students related to alcohol use and sexual assault (Testa et al. 2010), and alcohol policies (Lippy and DeGue 2014). My focus in this book on bystander behavior is not meant to suggest that these other components of prevention are not important. Indeed, sexual and relationship violence is a complex problem that will require multi-faceted responses (Banyard 2013, 2014).

This book draws from literature across forms of helping, types of interpersonal violence, and studies of attitude and behavior change. I try to highlight different points in the lifespan where training bystanders can be encouraged. We need prevention approaches that highlight the interconnections between forms of interpersonal violence (Banyard 2014; Hamby and Grych 2013). Too often our work focuses only on one. To date most bystander work, whether research on what promotes it or on prevention programs, use college student samples. Indeed, with the exception of Cook-Craig et al. (2014), Katz et al. (2011), Miller et al. (2013), and Potter and Moynihan (2011) most evaluations of bystander programs have been on university campuses. Currently, organizations, that focus on preventing child sexual abuse,such as Stop It Now!, are further adapting a bystander approach to teach adults how to be active bystanders to prevent child sexual abuse. The potential of a bystander approach is far reaching but has to date been hindered by an overly narrow focus on thin slices of an overall model of bystander action presented here.

2.6 Summary

- Bystanders are individuals who are present in situations in communities where there is risk for sexual assault or relationship abuse and by their presence have the potential to alter the outcome of the situation. They are individuals who are carriers of community norms related to SV and IPV and gatekeepers of resources and policies that effect response to SV and IPV. They are friends, family, co-workers of victims who are recipients of victims' disclosures.
- Bystanders can play a role at all levels of prevention: primary, secondary, and tertiary.
- Bystanders have powerful potential as prevention agents to address SV and IPV.

2.7 Implications for Practice

While the ultimate responsibility for sexual and relationship abuse rests with perpetrators of these acts, theories about the causes of sexual and relationship violence also point to the importance of witnesses or bystanders who are in positions to come to the aid of victims or interrupt risky situations. A number of promising prevention programs that train bystanders exist. They use formats that include in person educational workshops, social marketing campaigns, and online trainings. Empirical analyses of these programs show promising results for their effectiveness at changing attitude and increasing bystander action (Katz and Moore 2013). Much of the research on which our understanding of bystanders and the role, including what influences them to take action comes from looking at other behaviors—informal social control of rule violations like littering, helping someone who has dropped their books or who has a medical emergency. As described above, sexual and relationship abuse comprise a variety of behaviors (McMahon and Banyard 2011) some of which may involve low-cost helping behaviors but others of which may require moral courage—acts that have little apparent benefit to the bystander and may in fact carry negative consequences for him or her (Greitemeyer et al. 2006; Osswald et al. 2010). Educating community members to take action as responsive bystanders, then, requires motivating people to notice an array of situations and have ready a broad variety of actions they might take. We need to next examine research on bystanders and what factors influence behavior to see if the model for bystander focused prevention we are using is adequate. And if not, we need to revise these models and perhaps think differently about how best to promote safe bystander action so that we can be more effective in our prevention efforts.

References

Abbey, A., McAuslan, P., Zawacki, T., & Clinton, A. M. (2001). Attitudinal, experiential, and situational predictors of sexual assault perpetration. *Journal of Interpersonal Violence, 16*, 784–807.

Adams, D. (Sept. 3, 2013). http://www.boston.com/metrodesk/2013/09/03/prosecutors-say-somerville-high-school-teens-were-assaulted-with-broom-stick-one-suspect-held-for-dangerousness-hearing/stWcYQLg7y3YUuwzYJGelK/story.html

Ahrens, C. E., Rich, M. D., & Ullman, J. B. (2011). Rehearsing for real life: The impact of the InterACT sexual assault prevention program on self-reported likelihood of engaging in bystander interventions. *Violence Against Women, 17*, 760–776.

Anderson, L. A., & Whiston, S. C. (2005). Sexual assault education programs: A meta-analytic examination of their effectiveness. *Psychology of Women Quarterly, 29*, 374–388.

Banyard, V. L. (2011). Who will help prevent sexual violence: Creating an ecological model of bystander intervention. *Psychology of Violence: Special Issue on Theories of Violence, 1*, 216–229.

Banyard, V. L. (2013). Go big or go home: Reaching for a more integrated view of violence prevention. *Psychology of Violence, 3*, 115–120.

Banyard, V. L. (2014). Improving college campus based prevention of violence against women: A strategic plan for research built on multi-pronged practices and policies. *Trauma, Violence, and Abuse, 15*, 339–351.

Banyard, V. L., Moynihan, M. M., & Plante, E. G. (2007). Sexual violence prevention through bystander education: An experimental evaluation. *Journal of Community Psychology, 35*, 463–481.

Banyard, V., Weber, M., Grych, J., & Hamby, S. (in press). Where are the helpful bystanders? Ecological niche and victims' perceptions of bystander intervention. *Journal of Community Psychology*.

Boswell, A. A. Spade, J. Z. (1996). Fraternities and collegiate rape culture: Why are some fraternities more dangerous places for women?, *Gender & Society, 10*, 133–147.

Break the Cycle (2006) *Bystander Survey, 2006*. Opinion Research Corporation. http://www.breakthecycle.org/dating-violence-research/bystander-survey.

Brodsky, A. E. (1996). Resilient single mothers in risky neighborhoods: Negative psychological sense of community. *Journal of Community Psychology, 24*, 347–363.

Burke, S. (2015). Vanderbilt rape victim to other sexual violence victims "you are not alone." Huffington Post, Jan. 29, 2015.

Buzawa, E. S. & Austin, T. (1993). Determining police response to domestic violence victims. *The American Behavioral Scientist, 36*, 610–623.

Campbell, (1998). The community response to rape: Victims' experiences with the legal, medical, and mental health systems. *American Journal of Community Psychology, 26*, 355–379.

Campbell, et al. (2001). Preventing the "second rape:" rape survivors' experiences with community service provides. *Journal of Interpersonal Violence, 16*, 1239–1259.

Capaldi, D. M., KNoble, N. B., Shortt, J. W., & Kim, H. K. (2012). A systematic review of risk factors for intimate partner violence. *Partner Abuse, 3*, 231–280.

Centers for Disease Control Prevention. (2004). *Sexual violence prevention: beginning the dialogue*. Atlanta, GA: Centers for Disease Control and Prevention.

Chabot, H. F., Tracy, T. L., Manning, C. A., & Poisson, C. A. (2009). Sex, attribution, and severity influence intervention decisions of informal helpers in domestic violence. *Journal of Interpersonal Violence, 24*, 1696–1713.

Chaurand, N., & Brauer, M. (2008). What determines social control? People's reactions to counternormative behaviors in urban environment. *Journal of Applied Social Psychology, 38*, 1689–1715.

Chekroun, P., & Brauer, M. (2002). The bystander effect and social control behavior: The effect of the presence of others on people's reactions to norm violations. *European Journal of Social Psychology, 32*, 853–867.

CNN (2009). Accessed from http://www.cnn.com/2009/CRIME/10/27/california.gang.rape. investigation/

Cohen, N. (Nov. 24, 2014). 3 more Ramapo College students charged in campus sex assault, prosecutor says. Accessed from http://www.nj.com/bergen/index.ssf/2014/11/3_more_ramapo_college_students_charged_in_campus_sex_assault_prosecutor_says.html#incart_related_storiesstsstanders%20charged

Coker, A. L., Cook-Craig, P. G., Williams, C. M., Fisher, B. S., Clear, E. R., Garcia, L. S., & Hegge, L. M. (2011). Evaluating green dot: An active bystander intervention to reduce sexual assault on the college campuses. *Violence Against Women, 17*, 777–796.

Coker, A. L., Fisher, B. S., Bush, H. M., Swan, S. C., Williams, C. M., Clear, E. R., & DeGue, S. (2014). Evaluation of the green dot bystander intervention to reduce interpersonal violence among college students across three campuses. *Violence Against Women, 20*, 1179–1202.

Cook-Craig, P. G., Coker, A. L., Clear, E. R., Garcia, L. S., Bush, H. M., Brancato, C. J., et al. (2014). Challenge and opportunity in evaluating a diffusion-based active bystanding prevention program green dot in high schools. *Violence Against Women, 20*, 1179–1202.

Dahl (2013, March, 18) CBS News http://www.cbsnews.com/news/steubenville-rape-update-bystanders-coaches-and-parents-will-now-be-focus-of-ohio-ag-mike-dewine/

Dardis, C. M., Dixon, K. J., Edwards, K. M., & Turchik, J. A. (in press). A gendered examination of the factors related to dating violence perpetration and associated theoretical explanations: A review of the literature. *Trauma, Violence, and Abuse.*

Darley, J. M. & Latané, B. (1968). Bystander intervention in emergencies: Diffusion of responsibility. *Journal of Personality and Social Psychology, 8*, 377–383.

DeGue, S., Holt, M. K., Massetti, G. M., Matjasko, J. L., Tharp, A. T., & Valle, L. A. (2012). Looking ahead toward community-level strategies to prevent sexual violence. *Journal of Women's Health, 21*, 1–3.

DeGue, S., Valle, A., Holt, M. K., Massetti, G. M., Matjasko, J. L., & Tharp, A. T. (2014). A systematic review of primary prevention strategies for sexual violence perpetration. *Aggression and Violent Behavior, 19*, 346–362.

Edwards, K., Mattingly, M. J., Dixon. K. J., & Banyard, V. L. (2014). Community matters: Intimate partner violence among young adults. *American Journal of Community Psychology, 53*, 198–207.

Fabiano, P. M., Perkins, H. W., Berkowitz, A., Linkenbach, J., & Stark, C. (2003). Engaging men as social justice allies in ending violence against women: Evidence for a social norms approach. *Journal of American College Health, 52*, 105–112.

Ferrans, S. D., Selman, R. L., & Feigenberg, L. F. (2012). Rules of the culture and personal needs: Witnesses' decision-making processes to deal with situations of bullying in middle school. *Harvard Educational Review, 82*, 445–470.

Finkelhor, D., Vanderminden, J., Turner, H., & Hamby, S. (2014). Youth exposure to violence prevention programs in a national sample. *Child Abuse and Neglect, 38*, 677–686.

Foubert, J. D., & Newberry, J. T. (2006). Effects of two versions of an empathy-based rape prevention program on fraternity men's survivor empathy, attitudes, and behavioral intent to commit rape or sexual assault. *Journal of College Student Development, 47*, 133–148.

Frye, V. (2007). The informal social control of intimate partner violence against women: Exploring personal attitudes and perceived neighborhood social cohesion. *Journal of Community Psychology, 35*, 1001–1018.

Frye, V., Galea, S., Tracy, M., Bucciarelli, A., Putnam, S., & Wilt, S. (2008). The role of neighborhood environment and risk of intimate partner femicide in a large urban area. *American Journal of Public Health, 98*, 1473–1479.

Frye, V., Paul, M. M., Todd, M. J., Lewis, V., Cupid, M., Coleman, J., & O'Campo, P. (2012). Informal social control of intimate partner violence against women: Results from a concept mapping study of urban neighborhoods. *Journal of Community Psychology, 40*, 828–844.

Gidycz, C. A., & Dardis, C. M. (2014). Feminist self-defense and resistance training for college students: a critical review and recommendations for the future. *Trauma, Violence, and Abuse, 15*, 322–333.

Gidycz, C. A., Orchowski, L. A., & Berkowitz, A. D. (2011). Preventing sexual aggression among college men: An evaluation of a social norms and bystander intervention program. *Violence Against Women, 17*, 720–742.

Gonzalez, T. (2015). What happened in Vanderbilt dorm? Rape trial starts Monday. Usatoday.com

Gracia, E., Garcia, F., & Lila, M. (2009). Public responses to intimate partner violence against women: The influence of perceived severity and personal responsibility. *The Spanish Journal of Psychology, 12*, 648–656.

Greitemeyer, T., Fischer, P., Kastenmuller, A., & Frey, D. (2006). Civil courage and helping behavior: Differences and similarities. *European Psychologist, 11*, 90–98.

Hamby, S., & Grych, J. (2013). *The web of violence*. Springer, Berlin.

Hamby, S., Weber, M., Grych, J., & Banyard, V. (2015). What difference do bystanders make? The association of victim outcomes with bystander involvement in a community sample. *Psychology of Violence*, online first.

Harari, H., Harari, O., & White, R. V. (1985). The reaction to rape by American male bystanders *The Journal of Social Psychology, 125,*, 653–658.

Humphrey, S. E., & Kahn, A. S. (2000). Fraternities, athletic teams, and rape: Importance of identification with a risky group. *Journal of Interpersonal Violence, 15*, 1313–1322.

Katz, J. (1995). Reconstructing masculinity in the locker room: The mentors in violence prevention project. *Harvard Educational Review, 65*, 163–174.

Katz, J., Heisterkamp, A., & Flemming, A. M. (2011). The social justice roots of the mentors in violence prevention model and its application to a high school setting. *Violence Against Women, 17*, 684–702.

Katz, J., & Moore, J. (2013). Bystander education training for campus sexual assault prevention: an initial meta-analysis. *Violence and Victims, 28*, 1054–1067.

Kleinsasser, A., Jouriles, E. N., McDonald, R., & Rosenfield, D. (2015). An online bystander intervention program for the prevention of sexual violence. *Psychology of Violence, 5*, 227–235.

Knowledge Networks (2011). College dating violence and abuse poll. Accessed from https://www.breakthecycle.org/college-dating-violence-and-abuse-poll

Lee, H. K. (2015, February, 2). Ex-Stanford swimmer pleads no guilty to rape charges. Accessed from http://www.sfgate.com/bayarea/article/Ex-Stanford-swimmer-pleads-not-guilty-to-rape-6056929.php

Levine, M., Taylor, P.J., & Best, R. (2011) Third parties, violence, and conflict resolution the role of group size and collective action in the microregulation of violence *Psychological Science, 22*, 406-412

Lippy, C., & DeGue, S. (2014). Exploring alcohol policy approaches to prevent sexual violence perpetration. *Trauma, Violence, & Abuse. (Online first)*.

Lisak, D., & Miller, P. M. (2002). Repeat rape and multiple offending among undetected rapists. *Violence and Victims, 17*, 73–84.

Lonsway, K. A. (1996). Preventing acquaintance rape through education: What do we know? *Psychology of Women Quarterly, 20*, 229–265.

Lonsway, K. A., Banyard, V. L., Berkowitz, A. D., Gidycz, C. A., Katz, J. T., & Koss, M. P. (2009, January, 1–20). Rape prevention and risk reduction: Review of the research literature for practitioners. *VAWnet: The National Online Resource Center on Violence Against Women*. http://www.vawnet.org/sexual-violence/summary.php?doc_id_1655&find_type_web_desc_AR

Malik, S., Sorenson, S. B., & Aneshensel, C. S. (1997). Community and dating violence among adolescents: Perpetration and victimization. *Journal of Adolescent Health, 21*(5), 291–302.

McCauley, H. L., Tancredi, D. J., Silverman, J. G., Decker, M. R., Austin, S. B., McCormick, M. C., & Miller, E. (2013). Gender-equitable attitudes, bystander behavior, and recent abuse perpetration against heterosexual dating partners of male high school athletes. *American Journal of Public Health, 103*, 1882–1887.

McDonnell, K. A., Burke, J. G., Gielen, A. C., O'Campo, P., & Weidl, M. (2011). Women's perceptions of their community's social norms towards assisting women who have experienced intimate partner violence. *Journal of Urban Health: Bulletin of the New York Academy of Medicine, 88*, 240–253.

McMahon, S., & Banyard, V. L. (2012). When can I help? A conceptual framework for the prevention of sexual violence through bystander intervention. *Trauma, Violence, and Abuse, 13*, 3–14.

McMahon, S., Banyard, V., & McMahon, S. (2015). Incoming students' bystander behaviors to prevent sexual violence. *Journal of College Student Development, 56*, 488-493.

McMahon, S., Postmus, J. L., Warrener, C., & Koenick, R. A. (2014). Utilizing peer education theater for the primary prevention of sexual violence on college campuses. *Journal of College Student Development, 55*, 78–85.

Menning, C. L. (2009). Unsafe at any house? Attendees' perceptions of microlevel environmental traits and personal safety at fraternity and nonfraternity parties. *Journal of Interpersonal Violence, 24*, 1714–1734.

Miller, E., Tancredi, D. J., McCauley, H. L., Decker, M. R., Virata, M. C. D., Anderson, H. A., Stetkevich, N., Brown, E. W., Moideen, F., & Silverman, J. G. (2012). "Coaching boys into men": A cluster-randomized controlled trial of a dating violence prevention program. *Journal of Adolescent Health, 51*, 431–438.

O'Connell, M. E., Boat, T., & Warner, K. E. (Eds.). (2009). *Preventing mental, emotional, and behavioral disorders among young people: Progress and possibilities*. Washington, D.C.: The National Academies Press. National Research Council and Institute of Medicine of the National Academies.

Opinion Research Corporation. Accessed from www.loveisnotabuse.com/itstimetotalk

Osswald, S., Greitemeyer, T., Fischer, P., & Frey, D. (2010). What is moral courage? Definition, explication, and classification of a complex construct. In C. L. Purry & S. J. Lopez (Eds.), *The psychology of courage: Modern research on an ancient virtue*. Washington, D.C.: American Psychological Association.

Paul, L. A., & Gray, M. J. (2011). Sexual assault programming on college campuses: Using social psychological belief and behavior change principles to improve outcomes. *Trauma, Violence, & Abuse, 12*(2), 99–109.

Penner, L. A., Dovidio, J. F., Piliavin, J. A., & Schroeder, D. A. (2005). Prosocial behavior: Multilevel perspectives. *Annual Review of Psychology, 56*, 365–392.

Perkins, D. D., Meeks, J.W., & Taylor, R. B. (1992). The physical environment of street blocks and resident perceptions of crime and disorder: Implications for theory and measurement. *Journal of Environmental Psychology, 12*, 21–34.

Pinchevsky, G. M., & Wright, E. M. (2012). The impact of neighborhoods on intimate partner violence and victimization. *Trauma, Violence, & Abuse, 13*(2), 112–132.

Planty, M. (2002). *Third-party involvement in violent crime, 1993–1999*. Bureau of Justice Statistics Special Report. Washington, D.C. U.S. Department of Justice. NCJ189100.

Potter, S. J. (2012). Using a multimedia social marketing campaign to increase active bystanders on the college campus. *Journal of American College Health, 60*, 282–295.

Potter, S. J., & Moynihan, M. M. (2011). Bringing in the bystander in-person prevention program to a U.S. military installation: Results from a pilot study. *Military Medicine, 176*, 870–875.

Pozzoli, T., Gini, G., & Vieno, A. (2012). The role of individual correlates and class norms in defending and passive bystanding behavior in bullying: A multilevel analysis. *Child Development, 83*, 1917–1931.

Preston, J. (2013, March, 18). http://thelede.blogs.nytimes.com/2013/03/18/how-blogger-helped-steubenville-rape-case-unfold-online/?_php=true&_type=blogs&_r=0

Rogers, E. M. (2002). Diffusion of preventive innovations. *Addictive Behaviors, 27*, 989–993.

Rothman, E. F., Johnson, R. M., Young, R., Weinberg, J., Azrael, D., & Molnar, B. E. (2011a). Neighborhood-level factors associated with physical dating violence perpetration: Results of a representative survey conducted in Boston, MA. *Journal of Urban Health: Bulletin of the New York Academy of Medicine, 88*, 201–213.

References

Rothman, E. F., Johnson, R. M., Young, R., Weinberg, J., Azrael, D., & Molnar, B. E. (2011). Neighborhood-level factors associated with physical dating violence perpetration: Results of a representative survey conducted in Boston, MA. *Journal of Urban Health: Bulletin of the New York Academy of Medicine*. doi:10.1007/s11524-011-9543-z

Salazar, L. F., Vivolo-Kantor, A., Hardin, J., & Berkowitz, A. (2014). A web-based sexual violence bystander intervention for male college students: Randomized control trial. *Journal of Medical Internet Research, 16*, e203.

Salmivalli, C., Voeten, M., & Poskiparta, E. (2011). Bystanders matter: Associations between reinforcing, defending, and the frequency of bullying behavior in classrooms. *Journal of Clinical Child and Adolescent Psychology, 40*, 668–676.

Schwartz, M. D., & DeKeseredy, W. S. (1997). *Sexual assault on the college campus: The role of male peer support*. Thousand Oaks, CA: Sage.

Schwartz, M. D., DeKeseredy, W. S., Tait, D., & Alvi, S. (2001). Male peer support and a feminist routine activities theory: Understanding sexual assault on the college campus. *Justice Quarterly, 18*, 623–649.

Shernock, S. (2005). Third party roles in intimate partner violence incidents and their effects on police response in a statewide rural jurisdiction. *Journal of Police and Criminal Psychology, 20*, 22–39.

Shotland, R. L., & Straw, M. K. (1976). Bystander response to an assault: When a man attacks a woman. *Journal of Personality and Social Psychology, 34*, 990–999.

Snyder, J. A., Schererb, H. L., & Fisher, B. S. (2012). Social organization and social ties: Their effects on sexual harassment victimization in the workplace. *Work, 42*, 137–150.

Strang, E., & Peterson, Z. D. (2013). The relationships among perceived peer acceptance of sexual aggression, punishment certainty and sexually aggressive behavior. *Journal of Interpersonal Violence, 28*, 3369–3385.

Taylor, B. G., Stein, N. D., Mumford, E. A. & Woods, D. (2013). Shifting Boundaries: an experimental evaluation of a dating violence prevention program in middle schools, *Prevention science, 14*, 64–76.

Testa, M., Hoffman, J. H., Livingston, J. A., & Turrisi, R. (2010). Preventing college women's sexual victimization through parent based intervention: A randomized control trial. *Prevention Science, 11*, 308–318.

Tharp, A. T., DeGue, S., Valle, L. A., Brookmeyer, K. A., Massetti, G. M., & Matjasko, J. L. (2012). A systematic qualitative review of risk and protective factors for sexual violence perpetration. *Trauma, Violence, & Abuse, 14*, 133–167.

Twemlow, S. W., & Sacco, F. C. (2013). How and why does bystanding have such a startling impact on the architecture of school bullying and violence? *International Journal of Applied Psychoanalytic Studies, 10*, 289–306.

Ullman, S. (2010). *Talking about sexual assault: Society's response to survivors*. Washington, DC: American Psychological Association.

Vagi, K. J., Rothman, E. F., Latzman, N. E., Tharp, A T., Hall, D. M., & Breiding, M. J. (2013). Beyond correlates: a review of risk and protective factors for adolescent dating violence perpetration. *Journal of Youth and Adolescence, 42*, 633–649.

Weiss, H. E. (2011). Adolescents as a source of social control: The utility of adolescent social capital for reducing violent delinquency. *Sociological Spectrum, 31*, 554–578.

West, A., & Wandrei, M. L. (2002). Intimate partner violence a model for predicting interventions by informal helpers. *Journal of Interpersonal Violence, 17*, 972–986.

Wilson, J. Q. & Kelling, G. L. (Feb. 1982). Broken windows. *The Atlantic Monthly*, 29 38.

Winerip, M. (Feb. 7,2014). Stepping up to stop sexual assault. *The New York Times*. http://www.nytimes.com/2014/02/09/education/edlife/stepping-up-to-stop-sexual-assault.html

Chapter 3
Pieces of Bystander Action

> *I obviously didn't want to step in 'cause I didn't know them very well but I was like well this isn't right… And our other friends-basically they all knew what was going on and we were just kinda like well we don't know what to do.*
>
> *Cause she was just like 'I'm fine' and that's all she said. But she really didn't make eye-contact, so I felt really uncomfortable. I was just really concerned that there was something going on. It was just my automatic response that she might need help.*
>
> *I did it just because if I was in that situation, or if one of my friends was, I would want someone to tell me.*
> —College students speaking about being bystanders to sexual and relationship abuse

Abstract Variables that inhibit or facilitate bystander action are needed as the building blocks of our logic models and learning objectives for prevention curricula and tools. This chapter summarizes key empirical work about who takes action and under what circumstances. The who, what, where, when, and why of bystander actions are explored. The review draws from work on bystanders more broadly, as well as specific instances of bystander action to prevent violence. Strengths and limitations of this research for prevention practices and gaps in our understanding of bystander actions are described to set a context for the revised model of bystander action described later in the book.

Keywords Bystander behavior correlates · Helping · Altruism · Social ecological model

Looking across the research literature on bystander behavior we find a number of theories and empirical studies that explain helping and bystander action. Variables that inhibit or facilitate action become the building blocks of our logic models and learning objectives for prevention curricula and tools. However, to the extent these theories and research questions are limited; they may also restrict our impact. In this chapter I summarize key empirical literature about the who, what, where, and when of bystander action and helping. These factors include cognitions, emotions and intentions that make up bystander attitudes and influence a range of bystander behaviors, the "attitude system" of bystander intervention (Zimbardo and Leippe, 1991, p. 33). They also include important relational/social and contextual factors (Levine et al. 2012).

Each section begins with a review of the helping and bystander literature more broadly (including the study of helping in emergency situations, informal control of criminal or norm violating behavior including bullying, and the study of relationships) and then summarizes available findings that are more specific to sexual and relationship violence. In order to best organize this broad range of findings I draw from the social-ecological model of Bronfenbrenner (1977) that outlines many different levels at which variables may influence human behavior (factors within the individual, factors related to close relationships with family and peers, factors related to local settings including workplace, school, and community, and finally aspects of the wider society and culture) (see Banyard 2011 for a review and use of this framework to organize research on bystander intervention). I also use Flay et al. (2009) Theory of Triadic Influence that starts with the ecological model but goes beyond it as well.

Flay et al. sought to integrate different theories of health behavior change under one model, identifying different layers of variables that would pertain to any given health issue. This model begins with the Social Ecological Model, grouping causal factors under intra-personal, social-situational, and cultural environment/community headings (p. 455). Under these headings however, is a consideration of time, with some variables being farther away from the current decision to engage in a behavior like helping. These factors are what Flay et al. call "underlying causes and predisposing influences." These set the foundation for the behavior but are influences that were likely set in motion earlier in an individual's history. The best time to address these variables and shape the healthy outcomes we would like to see is when they are developing, through infancy and early childhood prevention work (for example via social emotional learning curricula that promote empathy and perspective taking; Durlak et al. 2011). Flay et al. also describe "proximal immediate predictors (p. 455)" that are the variables that affect behavioral choices more immediately in the moment including temporary situational characteristics. For example, being one of many bystanders in a large crowd leads to diffusion of responsibility and less bystander action (Latané and Darley 1970). In what follows in this chapter I try to indicate factors related to bystander action that are both distal and proximal and that span the ecological model.

Prevention is much easier to do with factors closer in time to when the attitudes or behaviors develop. That is, it is much easier to change something that is in the process of developing rather than a belief, behavior, etc. that has become an ingrained habit for an individual or community. Thus, considering the range of variables related to intervention can help us target different leverage points at different places in the lifespan. For example, bystander intervention for bullying among school children may work best when leveraging aspects of moral development that are part of what is developing at that point in the lifespan. Work with college students might need to instead harness motivations related to taking care of relationships, fitting in with peer norms, or forming an identity as a helpful person, developmental concerns for that age group that may be a better source of prevention motivation. This chapter dissects these distal and proximal factors in the small compartments of who, when, why, and where bystander actions occur.

3.1 Who

When asking the question about "who" in bystander intervention we can look both at who is the bystander—examining personal characteristics that may make them more or less likely to step in—and who is the person needing help—characteristics that may make receiving help more or less likely. Both have been the focus of research though most studied have been general characteristics of prosocial people with minimal attention to who is helped.

3.1.1 Who Helps?

3.1.1.1 Lessons from Helping in Contexts Other Than SV and IPV

There are several different layers to understanding who provides help. At the innermost layer, evolutionary theories and research on biological and genetic foundations of helping suggest that the foundation of helping behavior may be hardwired, particularly via empathy (Penner et al. 2005) suggesting both that all individuals have the capacity to help and that biology may explain some of the variation we see in how much people help others. Carlo and colleagues (Carlo and Randall 2002; Carlo et al. 1999; Eisenberg et al. 1999, 2002) define helping as related to personality, what they call "prosocial tendencies." These aspects of helpful or prosocial behavior begin in childhood and are somewhat stable into early adulthood. Planned forms of helping (volunteering or watching a neighbor's house or planning in advance to give a friend a ride) showed modest and mixed correlations with personality traits like social responsibility and mastery, though not for all samples (Amato 1990). In the context of bullying, personality measures like empathy, extroversion and openness were related to different types of bystander action (Freis and Gurung 2013). Working for social justice such as challenging racism (a form of looking out for others) has been linked to the openness dimension of the Big Five (Osswald et al. 2010). Studies have supported the idea that increased empathy is related to greater helping and tha at bystander's physical strength is also a factor (Coke et al. 1978; Fischer et al. 2011).

Demographic characteristics are also part of this intra-individual layer of influences. Other reviews highlight personal demographics like gender (Banyard 2011; Eagley and Crowley 1986; George et al. 1998). For example, gender scripts influenced the types of actions men and women chose with men more likely to help in heroic, assertive and public ways and women more likely to help through nurturing and caring in social networks. The result of this study was that while overall, men and women did not differ in the amount of helping they did, they were different in when they helped, with each gender more likely to help in circumstances congruent with gender role beliefs (Carlo and Randall 2002; Dovidio et al. 2006; Eagly 2009). What is more, research also suggests that correlates of helping behavior vary by gender and that different aspects of masculinity affect confidence about intervening and concerns about negative outcomes of bystander action (Carlson 2008; George et al. 1998; Leone et al. 2015). The gender of an individual bystander also intersects with the gender of other present bystanders (Levine and Crowther 2008) such that men are more likely to intervene when other bystanders are women and women are less likely to help in the presence of men, likely due to activation of internal gender scripts about women needing help and men seeing their role as leaders even in helping situations.

Personal experiences with an issue also impact action. More highly educated community members and those in roles where they might come in contact with child maltreatment were more likely to take action to address suspected child neglect (Fledderjohann and Johnson 2012). Individuals who have experienced trauma or victimization themselves are also more likely to help others (Christy and Voigt 1994; Frazier et al. 2013). On the other hand, a study of IPV specifically found those with personal experience were less likely to take bystander action by reporting to police (Gracia and Herrero 2006).

More consistent results have been found for moral development and coping as correlates of defending behavior for bullying. Bystanders who stepped in to help peers who were being bullied rather than passively standing by scored higher on an assessment of moral responsibility (this was particularly true for adolescent samples) and used more problem-focused coping (rather than distancing or internalizing coping strategies) (Caravita et al. 2012; Pozzoli and Gini 2010). Studies on moral courage (instances when individuals step in to address human rights and other social justice issues rather than just more low-cost helping instances) showed participants who had anger at injustice and strong ethical standards and sense of moral justice (Osswald et al. 2010). These studies have in common a focus on internal and rather stable qualities of an individual that may impact their likelihood of helping others. They are distal variables that shape the lens through which key intentions, attitudes, cognitions, and emotions more proximal to helping are filtered (Zimbardo and Leippe 1991). They may best be part of the focus of prevention and youth development work early on.

There are also a constellation of attitudes that research shows are linked to bystander actions. These include self-efficacy and sense of responsibility. Latané and Darley's (1970) classic research on the bystander effect was grounded in the notion that individuals in larger groups experience "diffusion of responsibility" that works against taking action. Bystanders in large groups felt others would step in instead. Furthermore, research consistently shows that people who feel more confident in their ability to help are more likely to do so.

3.1.1.2 Lessons from Research on SV and IPV

Similar patterns of factors at the individual level have also been found for bystanders to SV and IPV including gender, personal experiences and attitudes. For example, self-efficacy is linked to greater bystander action related to SV and IPV (Banyard 2011; Lazarus & Signal, 2013). As with helping more generally, some studies find gender differences in how men and women indicate they will take action in situations of SV and IPV (Chabot et al. 2009; Nicksa 2010, 2014). More nuanced measures of constructs like masculinity show that men who believe in gender norms about it being important for men to be strong and tough had greater concerns about negative consequences for stepping in as a bystander to SV. Men who believed that it is important for men to be respected by others reported greater bystander confidence (Leone et al. 2015). Indeed, aspects of gender role stress as assessed in this study were related to different relationships between traditionally studied bystander variables like confidence and perceived pros and cons for intervention. Women were more confident about the helpfulness of the support they provided to a friend who told them about an unwanted sexual experience, though they also reported feeling more emotional distress than men, and were more likely to endorse helpful responses to IPV survivors (Ahrens and Campbell 2000; Banyard et al. 2011; Beeble et al. 2008; West and Wandrei 2002). Studies show that personal experiences with child maltreatment of IPV were related to greater bystander action or intent in some studies (Chabot et al. 2009; Frye 2007) but not others (Gracia and Herrero 2006) with differences likely due to the type of bystander action being assessed. This is relevant to understanding gender since men and women have different risk of exposure to various types of interpersonal violence across the lifespan.

Attitudes specific to SV and IPV are also important for bystander action in these contexts. College students with greater sense of confidence or efficacy in themselves as helpful bystanders had greater intention to intervene and reported greater levels of bystander action (Banyard and Moynihan 2011), though gender also intersected with attitudes as woman displayed greater knowledge about sexual assault and lower acceptance of myths about rape (e.g., Suarez and Gadalla 2010; West and Wanderei 2002). In a community sample from an international study, willingness to report IPV was associated with lower tolerance of IPV (Gracia and Herrero 2006). Indicators of different stages of readiness to change, especially awareness and sense of responsibility related to sexual and relationship violence were related to bystander intentions and behaviors (Banyard et al. 2010; Banyard and Moynihan 2011; Gracia et al. 2009). Importantly, bystander prevention with young adults seems to increase efficacy for addressing sexual and relationship violence (Banyard et al. 2007; Cares et al. 2015).

3.1.2 Who Is Helped?

The "who" of helping and bystander action also requires us to ask who is helped? Interpersonal violence presents complicated situations where both victims and perpetrators can be the receivers of bystander action. Further, the person at whom the bystander action is directed could be a friend or stranger. We know that more general pro-social helping behavior is more likely to be provided to friends and family than strangers (Amato 1990; Penner et al. 2005), yet laboratory studies of bystander intervention usually use strangers as research confederates who help to stage the helping dilemma. To what extent does this make a difference in the barriers and facilitators of action? For example, studies of hypothetical crimes found bystanders less likely to report crimes when they knew the perpetrator (Nicksa 2014). Another vignette study found female college students had more intention to help children while men were more likely to help women (Laner et al. 2001).

3.1.3 Perpetrators Versus Victims

Nearly all of the psychological literature on bystanders has been about understanding help provided to those who need it. The outcome variable in research studies has been whether help was provided to someone having a medical emergency, stepping in to an argument, or offering instrumental help. For example, the arousal cost reward model of helping explains how the emotional arousal created when someone needs help compels us to take action on their behalf (Dovidio et al. 1991, 2006). This research is most relevant to helping victims. Thus, most of the research summarized in this chapter focuses on assisting potential victims. For example, rape myth acceptance, one indicator of victim blaming attitudes, was associated with lesser intent to help as a bystander (McMahon 2010). Perceptions of greater danger to a person in need also facilitated helping across studies (Fischer et al. 2006, 2011). Other researchers have described instances of moral courage, situations that differ from ordinary helping because there is a higher than normal chance that the bystander will experience negative consequences from their actions (a term that me be appropriate for understanding situations where there is risk for SV or IPV), anger seems to be a particularly activating emotion.

On the other hand, social control research in sociology is concerned with how communities as a whole respond to criminal behavior or deviance and express disapproval (Charuand and Brauer 2008). This theory seems most germane to interventions to address the perpetrator. Some similar and some different variables have been researched in this context. Social control is related to how a bystander thinks and feels about what they observe: how much do they see the behavior of the other person as deviant? How much do they see themselves as responsible for doing something about it? How legitimate do they think it is to exercise informal social control? How much does the behavior affect their own self interest—to what extent are they personally affected or harmed? How important is the norm that is being violated (some people may get more upset about environmental issues like littering or not picking up dog waste while others are more angered by hygiene issues like spitting)? How much does the situation bring up feelings of anger or disgust/distain? Higher levels of these thoughts and emotions are related to greater indications of willingness to exert social control against the person violating the social norm via deviant behavior.

3.1.4 Friends Versus Strangers/Ingroup Versus Outgroup

3.1.4.1 General Helping Situations

In the general bystander literature and work specific to sexual violence, people are more likely to help friends than strangers (Amato 1990; Bennett et al. 2014; Katz et al. 2014). Levine and colleagues have looked beyond the distinction between friends and strangers to what happens with bystander action if victims are in-group or out-group members. Even unknown victims who are perceived as in group members (e.g. fans of the same sports team or sport, part of the same campus) are more likely to be helped (Levine et al. 2005; Levine and Crowther 2008). This suggests that how the status of the person in need of help is perceived by the bystander can be influenced by information or framing from the social context. Levine and colleagues have discussed this in terms of social identity theory—that how we see our membership in groups and the connection of victims and perpetrators to those groups influences actions in both general helping and in situations where fighting occurs (Levine et al. 2012).

Interestingly, there may also be different barriers to helping friends and strangers. One study of helping in a sexual assault situation showed that sense of responsibility increased action to help strangers but was unrelated to helping friends. Further, feeling uncertain about the helping skills you have was a barrier to helping strangers but not a barrier to bystander intervention with friends (Bennett et al. 2014). Another study found greater sense of responsibility and empathy to help friends in a SV party vignette and these variables explained participants' greater likelihood of helping friends compared to strangers. Perceived barriers such as victim blaming attitudes and concerns about what others might think about a bystander stepping in did not seem to differ by whether the person needing help was a friend or stranger Katz et al. (2014). As noted above, intent to help varies by who the bystander knows (Bennett and Banyard 2014; Nicksa 2014). Correlates of each may be different and empirical models to date seem to do better at explaining factors related to helping strangers.

3.1.4.2 The Case of Violence

A complication in the case of SV and IPV is that frequently bystanders know both victims and perpetrators, and victims and perpetrators may also know each other. For example, individuals who overheard a potential relationship abuse situation were less likely to offer help if they believed the man and woman knew each other (Shotland and Straw 1976). In one study of two vignettes of a hypothetical sexual assault, college students were more likely to identify the situation as a problem if they knew the victim and less likely to label the situation as a problem if they knew the perpetrator. However, participants felt safer taking action if they knew either the victim or perpetrator compared to a situation involving strangers (Bennett and Banyard 2014). Participants had the greatest intent to intervene using tactics that both helped the victim and confronted the perpetrator when they only knew the victim. Participants who knew only the perpetrator in the scenario had lower intent to provide help to the victim, indicated greater intent to confront the perpetrator, and lower intent to contact outside resources (Bennett et al. 2015).

3.2 What or How

3.2.1 Lessons Learned from General Helping and Informal Social Control

A key piece of bystander action is having the skills to help (Burn 2009; Latané and Darley 1970). What then do bystander skills and actions consist of? How is it that bystanders intervene? Research is clear that both intent to take action (an attitude) and the actual action itself (behavior) are important components of bystander intervention. Behaviors have been assessed among bystanders in a number of ways. Social psychology most often uses laboratory studies. A confederate poses as someone in need of help. Bystanders are brought into the situation under the pretense of filling out surveys or some other behavior and an observer notes whether the bystander takes action to help the confederate. Describing the type of action taken is usually not the focus of study or only a small set of helping behaviors are called for by the situation (helping to fix a flat tire, helping to pick up dropped items). Nonetheless, different classifications of helping exist. For example, Amato (1990) distinguished between planned and spontaneous helping and found different correlates of each. Moral courage has been described as its own type of altruism distinct from helping. It involves addressing injustice and assisting people who face discrimination and unfair treatment because of less powerful social status. In these situations taking action may have high costs for the person who steps in and little personal benefit (for example, individuals who helped Jews in Nazi Germany or someone who steps in to defend a gay man who is being physically harassed for his sexual orientation) (Osswald et al. 2010). Practitioners in bystander prevention have created the "3 D's" to describe general categories of bystander action as direct action, distracting, or delegating (GreenDot, Etc. 2015).

3.2.2 Considering the Specifics of SV and IPV

Bystander intervention in the case of sexual and relationship violence is nearly always spontaneous and less amenable to the lab studies used most frequently in other studies of helping and prosocial behavior more generally (Banyard et al. 2014;

McMahon and Banyard 2011). Several methods have been used to try to document bystander action to address SV and IPV. Harari et al. (2001) were able to stage a sexual assault in a parking lot and observe whether bystanders stepped in to help. They operationalized helping minimally—as either approaching the couple, seeking out a policeman nearby or walking away with no intervention. Parrott et al. (2012) have developed an interesting lab model of sexual aggression where individuals were bystanders in the lab and observed decisions about showing a woman in another room sexually explicit media against her wishes. Speaking up against this behavior was measured as the bystander action. This is one of the few ways to date that seeks to assess bystander action for sexual or relationship violence directly.

Most bystander research uses self-report measures that describe a variety of actions across a continuum of situations (Banyard et al. 2014; McMahon and Banyard 2011). These actions can be direct within the situation (such as interrupting someone taking an intoxicated person away from a college party and up to their room or directly talking to a victim and trying to connect them with resources) or more indirect (enlisting friends to take someone home from a bar or encouraging friends of a victim to reach out to offer support) (Berkowitz 2009).

A study of teens found that most who had a friend in a violent relationship offered some sort of help and support, with talking to friends and offering advice or suggestions or encouraging their friend to leave the relationship being most common (Fry et al. 2013). A community sample of neighborhood residents' bystander actions related to intimate partner violence found several clusters or dimensions of helping including strategies focused on victims, focused on perpetrators, focused on neighborhoods or on formal helping systems (Frye et al. 2012). Community members reported differences in how possible it would be for them to prevent partner violence, reporting it would be easiest for them to provide help to victims or to access formal services (Frye et al. 2012). Preliminary studies found that factors related to different types of bystander action may vary but little research has explored or described these patterns (Banyard and Moynihan 2011). Thus, we do not yet know whether we need to teach different things to promote actions in low risk versus high risk situations or to encourage supportive behaviors toward victims. For example, Slater et al. (2013) found that in-group members were more likely to use more direct and confronting strategies to break up a fight while out-group members relied more heavily on trying to diffuse the situation with comments.

A number of challenges exist when trying to understand types of bystander action for SV and IPV. It is difficult to separate descriptions of the situation (at a party where someone's personal space is being violated versus hearing catcalls shouted from a passing car to a woman on the street) from types of bystander response as they are linked. Researchers often measure both at the same time, making it difficult to clearly summarize what we know about the "what" of bystander intervention as distinct from the "when" (a topic considered in more detail in the next section). We also know little about what actions are most helpful. This is a key question for prevention education as it would help us focus resources on skill building for the most effective and safe responses to sexual and relationship abuse. Planty (2002) indicated that victims most often reported that bystanders to crime made the situation better but few studies have investigated this question. Hamby et al. (2015) found that the helpfulness of bystanders varied by victimization type. What is more, whether a victim perceived the bystander to be helpful or not was more important in the link between bystanders and better victim outcomes that just whether or not a bystander was present. Bystander safety was also associated with more positive victim outcomes. So it is not just about whether a bystander takes action. It is also about what bystanders do, how what they do is perceived by the victim, and whether bystanders are themselves hurt in the process (Hamby et al. 2015). This is another critical component of the "what" of bystander intervention that has been under researched.

3.3 When

In order to describe when bystanders intervene I consider several topics. The first is describing the types of situations that constitute sexual and relationship abuse. Next we need to consider opportunity, an understudied topic in bystander research—to what extent do individuals find themselves in situations where they have the chance to help? Finally, I review literature about the nature of the situation—its status as a perceived emergency or not, for example. These are key proximal factors for bystander action no matter when an individual encounters it in the lifespan. In this area there is a growing base of research specific to SV and IPV and thus that is the bulk of the literature on which I draw except when noted.

3.3.1 Considering the Type of Situation

A number of factors impact when people step in to help and using the theory of triarchic influence most of these are more proximal, situational perceptions. These include whether the situation involves an emergency, perceptions of danger to those in need of help, as well as the presence and number of bystanders in the situation.

3.3.1.1 Notes from the Study of Prosocial Behavior More Broadly

As noted in earlier sections of this book, research related to bystander action spans several categories of behavior. Osswald et al. (2010) and Greitemeyer et al. (2006) distinguished between instances where helping is needed and instances of moral courage. Helping involves instances where there are likely few negative social consequences while moral courage are situations where action is needed but there is little potential benefit to the bystander and potentially many negative consequences. An accident or medical emergency is an example of helping while stepping in to challenge someone who is racially harassing someone is more about moral courage (Greitemeyer et al. 2006). Participants in several studies were asked to describe either a time when they helped or not or exhibited moral courage or not and then answered questions about correlates of this action or inaction. When looking at correlates of action separately for helping and courage, helping was significantly associated with greater empathy and quickness in perceiving a need. Both helping and courage actions were related to greater awareness of an emergency. Courage but not helping actions were related to greater felt responsibility, felt anger, perception of norms, and feeling one had skills to take action. These correlates reflect more distally developed variables like empathy and those more specific to the immediate situation like emotional reactions and norms.

3.3.1.2 The Complexity of Situations of SV and IPV

Sexual and relationship abuse span a number of different types of situations, and each of these types often unfold over time. Some instances where bystanders help with SV and IPV may look more like what Osswald et al. call helping but other instances are more clearly about moral courage. What is more, bystanders have the chance to take action before, during, or after an assault (McMahon and Banyard 2011). Bystanders might step in when they notice an escalation of risk factors, they might step in when an assault is taking place, they may choose to help after an assault, when a survivor seeks support or assistance or when a perpetrator discusses his actions. Most researched is how friends, family and professional helpers (law enforcement, advocates, medical and mental health professionals) respond when victims come forward to disclose what happened to them (Campbell et al. 1999; Fry et al. 2012; Ullman 2010). It is clear from this work that victims receive an array of both positive/supportive responses but also negative victim blaming comments and that negative responses in particular can increase a victim's distress after an assault. We know most of this from the perspective of victims who are clear about the importance of being believed, encouraged, and helped to find resources. We know much less about what enables bystanders to provide these responses at each of these more specific time points.

We also need to explore more about how taking action to help may need to differ between SV and IPV. For example, interviews with friends and family members of IPV survivors documented the long process involved with trying to support these individuals through abusive relationships that may go on for years and periods of leaving and reconnecting (Latta and Goodman 2011). Indeed, what survivors find helpful from bystanders may change depending on their own perceptions of the relationship they are in Edwards et al. (2012). The challenges of engagement and disengagement for bystanders may look different in instances of sexual violence that do not occur within the context of a long-term relationship. Support may need to be more short term and immediate but may need to include interfacing with different services systems and resources as a survivor seeks medical attention and makes choices about pressing criminal charges. Bystanders are also allocated different levels of responsibility for intervention related to these problems. In the case of child maltreatment, bystanders are often mandatory reporters who need to advise authorities as part of their actions. This has also become the case for "responsible employees" on college campuses [faculty and staff who are required under new Title IX provisions to alert campus authorities so that an investigation can be pursued (White House Task Force to Protect Students from Sexual Assault, 2014, notalone.gov)]. In Vermont all citizens are required to report instances of physical danger.

3.3.2 Understanding Opportunity to Intervene

Researchers have begun to study opportunity as its own aspect of bystander intervention. To some extent, this presents a methodological puzzle in that measuring how much helping someone does has to be put in the context of how much opportunity they have to take action (McMahon et al., in press). Studies showed that college students, for example, often reported high levels of opportunity to take action against sexual and relationship abuse (McMahon et al. 2015). More specifically, first year students reported having many chances to take action in low risk situations such as when someone was making harassing comments. Once opportunity was accounted for, college students were most likely, however, to actually take action in high risk situations where they worried an assault might be about to occur and least likely to take action proactively when given the chance to learn more about sexual violence and how it can be prevented [McMahon et al. 2015, in press]. Among a community sample of adults over 40% reported observing child neglect during the past year (Fledderjohann and Johnson 2012). Thus, research suggests that opportunities to be an active bystander to violence are plentiful.

3.3.3 Numbers of Other Bystanders

The classic work of Latané and Darley (1970) showed that bystanders were less likely to help when additional bystanders were present, what they termed the "bystander effect." They described several attitudes that influence this inaction. Diffusion of responsibility refers to a bystander feeling less motivation to step in when many other bystanders are present. Any one individual feels that others could step in which reduces any one person's motivation to do so. A second process is "evaluation apprehension." This attitude leaves bystanders concerned about how others' will see them if they take some sort of public action. Bystanders may be worried about making a mistake or doing something that others will judge negatively. As a result, bystanders may choose to do nothing in the presence of others, a construct that Latané and Nida also referred to as "audience inhibition" (Fischer et al. 2011; Latané and Nida 1981). Finally, there is the concept of "pluralistic ignorance" whereby bystanders who see others doing nothing, infer that those other bystanders do not see the situation as a problem and thus adopt this view themselves, reducing their sense that something needs to be done (Fischer et al. 2011; Latané and Nida 1981). This work reminds us that whether or not bystanders step in has to do with both the bystander and the people around him or her, proximal aspects of the situation.

Other work says its not just about the numbers but about the composition of the crowd. Levine and Crowther (2008) explored how gender roles can promote and hinder pro-social responses to both hypothetical vignettes and actual need for help. Across a series of studies they used both an imagined scenario of a man attacking a women and a staged opportunity for participants to actually provide help to a research confederate who posed as someone upset and needing support. While both men and women were exposed to the same situation where helping was needed, they varied the gender composition of the group of bystanders surrounding the research participant. They found that men increased helping when other bystanders were women while women decreased their helping when other bystanders were men. Levine and Crowther hypothesized that the results were due to the operation of gender norms such that women deferred to men in a group, assigning them more responsibility to help because of stereotypes about male assertiveness or heroism. Men in the presence of female bystanders responded to these same gender role beliefs and assumed leadership for providing help. Women were more likely to help in same-sex groups. In another study using innovative methods, coding CCTV footage of public aggression, researchers were able to document how third parties were able to lessen violence and aggression and how it was collaborative groups of bystanders rather than individuals who were successful at this suggesting the importance of bystanders responding when others could also be enlisted to help (Levine et al. 2011).

3.3.4 Perceptions of Emergency and Danger

Research on bystander intervention more generally finds that individuals are more likely to intervene if they identify the situation as more of an emergency. An important factor is whether the situation is dangerous just to the victim or to victim and others including bystanders. Bystanders are more likely to step in when they also feel at risk. In these circumstances they are also more likely to enlist others to help and more likely to see situation as a problem that needs to be addressed (Fischer et al. 2011). This may be because dangerous emergencies create a great deal of arousal (anxiety, concern, stress) that motivates bystanders to work with others to more effectively help to reduce the danger including potential costs to themselves (Fischer et al. 2006, 2011). More specific to SV and IPV is the variable of severity. Research finds greater intent to intervene in more severe situations (Bennett et al. 2015) though Gracia et al. (2009) did not find an effect for severity. People who think IPV happens often in a community, a potential marker of perceived severity, were more likely to report IPV positively (Gracia and Herrero 2006).

3.3.5 Perceived Barriers to Bystander Action

People engage in a costs/benefits analysis when deciding when to help. Social psychologists have described this in terms of "rational choice," that we choose the option that has the best outcomes (Paternotte 2011). Thus, bystander research has also catalogued barriers to intervention (Bennett et al. 2014; Burn 2009). These barriers include not being aware of the situation or not labeling it as a problem, and being concerned that the costs of action will be too high (either because of physical safety concerns or because of concerns that others will not support bystander action). It can also be the case that bystanders lack confidence or lack skills to know what to do. In one qualitative study of college students the following quotes were common:

> "it was difficult because it wasn't clear what was happening at first. I'd never been in a situation like that before. I just didn't know what to do so I was just kind of freaking out."
>
> "I was shocked and didn't know what to do and couldn't believe that something like that would happen to someone I've known almost my entire life"
>
> "I was like, this is a big problem, I don't know what to do and I didn't want to confront him to his face because he was very drunk and quite large"

One understudied aspect of barriers to intervention is the use of substances including alcohol. While a large volume of research links alcohol and sexual assault and alcohol use is also a risk factor for IPV, studies are relatively absent about how alcohol may make bystander action more or less likely. Some studies from the substance field may be useful here as they look at factors related to taking action or not related to friends who are drinking too much. This research that found that negative social norms (that is, social norms that promoted drinking as a positive behavior) were related to lower intentions to intervene related to alcohol use (Mollen et al. 2013). In the sexual assault field, research is clear that victim blame is higher and perpetrator blame less if the victim has been drinking, and these factors may lessen bystander action (Bieneck and Krahe 2011). Anecdotally, in my own work, participants who are young and on college campuses discussed their concerns about being an active bystander if they were underage and had been drinking, concerned that they would be punished for their own behavior if formal helpers were involved in the situation. This suggests alcohol use by perpetrators may lessen bystander actions. On the other hand, given what we know about the effects of alcohol on cognitions and decision making, it may also be the case that alcohol use may make bystanders themselves more likely to disregard their own safety and step in or perhaps to make different decisions about how to intervene. Though not specific to SV or IPV, a recent study used focus groups with community members who were part of community night life at the bars and pubs in the UK (Levine et al. 2012). These are social contexts in which alcohol is heavily involved. Yet participants described systems of bystander action and informal social control that operated in those contexts. This suggests that alcohol use, a risk factor for aggression that may require bystander action, does not interfere with some systems of informal social control by bystanders (Koelsch et al. 2012; Levine et al. 2012).

3.4 Why

Closely tied to when is why bystanders help. Classic social psychology research on bystanders focused more on what proximal conditions make action more or less likely rather than unpacking the motives of those who take action. There are some theories in the broader helping and altruism literature that speak to this question and researchers on bullying among children have offered hypotheses as well. Using the theory of triarchic influence, these variables are more distal to the bystander action performed—they involve aspects of individual motivation that likely develop early in the lifespan.

In studies of bullying among children, researchers described individual motives for helping in terms of moral responsibility. Girls who defended others against bullies showed higher or more developed ethical reasoning skills (Caravita et al. 2012). Researchers studying prosocial behavior more generally discuss more evolutionary motivations to help promote one's own and one's family and ingroups' survival (Penner et al. 2005 for a review). These are more distal factors, traits that need to be nurtured in early relational environments (Biglan et al. 2012). This work suggests that we need to begin building bystanders early in the lifespan (Carlo et al. 1999, 2003). Given recent research that shows many youth have been exposed to violence prevention messages (Finkelor et al. 2014) it will be interesting to see how children who get early bullying bystander prevention are primed to receive messages later about bystander behavior and sexual and relationship violence. To date we do not have answers to how these more distal experiences impact actions later on.

In between these distal motivations and more proximal variables described below, is why we help because of relationship oriented motivations of reciprocity and commitment (which in part explains why there is greater helping provided to friends) (Zimbardo and Leippe 1991 for a review). We help others so that they will help us in return later. In our quest to be accepted by others, we observe how they act and try behaviors we have seen others do (Fabiano et al. 2003; Stein 2007; Penner et al. 2005 for a review). Thus, part of why we help is because we see others who have stature within our community or sub-community modeling and endorsing helping attitudes and behaviors (Kelly 2004). This has been studied in terms of our perceptions of what we think others are doing (descriptive norms) and what we think others think we all should be doing (injunctive norms). Such norms can have a powerful impact on what we think and do (Fabiano et al. 2003;

Paul and Gray 2011) and some social marketing campaigns that aim to model positive social norms have shown success in changing attitudes that support bystander action to address SV and IPV (Potter and Stapleton 2012). Bystanders are motivated to act if they feel others share similar views. Research shows that norms affect attributions of blame to victims of IPV and one study found greater intent to help a victim of IPV after exposure to pro-helping norms, while decreases in intent to help were found after exposure to anti-helping norms (Baldri and Pagliaro 2014). Further, researchers in the communication field highlight how individual differences in the communication strategies people choose when trying to influence others come from variations in judgements about what constitutes effective communication styles. Differences in past relationships (a distal variable) and variations in immediate goals related to communication affect these varied perceptions (White & Malkowski, 2014). This work reminds us that a key component of understanding the "why" of bystander responses is to more carefully observe the motives or goals that may drive a bystander's selection of one communication or action strategy over another. More research on this topic is needed.

Peer norms are a part of this story as well. In the bullying literature, defenders of victims selected friends who were similar to them and that may have helped promote bystander action (Ruggieri et al. 2013) and classrooms where students perceived that teachers condemned bullying and thought it was a problem had lower rates of bullying and greater defending behavior (Hektner and Swenson 2012; Pozzoli et al. 2012; Sapouna et al. 2010; Veenstra et al. 2014). Among college students peer norms in favor of taking action against sexual violence were not related to greater bystander action overall, though it was related to great intent to help. However, there was a link between more positive norms and greater behavior among subgroups of students, particularly among Black men in college (Brown et al., in press). The role of peer norms and relationship variables will be discussed in more detail in Chap. 5 where I consider how to create change among bystanders. Interestingly, in a community sample in Spain, people who reported exposure to greater public discussion of IPV were more positive about reporting it (Gracia and Herrero 2006).

One theory that addresses more proximal variables related to motivation is the Arousal Cost Reward Model of helping (Dovidio et al. 1991, 2006). Emotional arousal is a source of motivation. Seeing someone in distress causes an uncomfortable level of emotional arousal. People are motivated to reduce uncomfortable arousal and will help others as a way of doing this if the costs are not higher than the benefits. There is empirical support for this model, though other researchers found emotions like love are linked to greater helping then distress or feeling solidarity (Lamy et al. 2012). Aspects of the situation can also influence access to different thoughts and some researchers have found playing prosocial video games of listening to prosocial music increases prosocial thoughts which are a mediating link to actually doing more helping (Greitemeyer and Osswald 2007, 2011).

3.5 Where

3.5.1 Cultural and Geographic Variability: The Potential Importance of Ecological Niche

Bystander behavior also occurs within a broader community context, what we might think about as ecological niches. We know that proximal situational factors like the presence of other bystanders impacts when someone will take action but to what extent do more distal setting characteristics have an impact on helping? These may be objective measures of the setting (rural versus urban) or perceptions of community cohesion, belonging, collective efficacy or they may be aspects of the cultural values a community holds. Understanding how helping differs by ecological niche may help us to better adapt and translate prevention tools to motivate bystander action in these different locations. To answer these questions researchers on prosocial helping more generally have compared helping rates across countries and across rural and urban settings. Relatively little of this work has been done related to SV and IPV specifically.

One way that communities differ from each other is in their physical characteristics and social processes. For example, one international study found less general, low-cost helping (when someone dropped a pen, when someone hurt themselves, or when a blind person needed help crossing a street) in wealthier countries (Levine et al. 2001) while another study focused on the crime of pick pocketing found more bystander intervention in a more advantaged community (Zhong 2010). More specific to IPV, community-level poverty was unrelated to bystander action, though at the level of individual income, more well to do individuals were less likely to help. Characteristics of the setting, such as poverty level, may matter mainly because of the perceptions and relationships that are affected within the community. Pinchevsky and Wright (2012) discussed how communities with high levels of economic disadvantage and where people move around a lot created the conditions for low collective efficacy, low social capital, and less communication. People were struggling to survive and had little time or energy for working on common goals with community members. Residential instability makes building relationships harder, though studies have been mixed with regard to whether community social processes like collective efficacy are related to perpetration rates and bystander intervention (Edwards et al. 2014; Frye 2007; Rothman et al. 2011). Recently, across different communities and different types of interpersonal violence, variables like collective efficacy, cohesion and trust in community authorities were related to greater bystander action or willingness to help (Edwards et al. 2014; Fledderjohann and Johnson 2012). Greater community support and collective efficacy were related to victims' perceiving bystanders as helpful and more safe (Banyard et al., in press).

Rural and urban differences have been found in helping, with greater altruistic behavior in rural communities (Rushton 1978), though others did not see an impact of city size on helping (Levine et al. 2001). Studies of SV and IPV have considered the unique challenges for survivors in rural communities but I could locate no studies that specifically compared urban and rural communities on bystander action to address IPV and SV. This may be an important direction for future research.

Culture, both in terms of race and ethnicity but also in terms of sets of values of different groups of people is yet another way that location or niche may matter for bystander intervention (Ferrans et al. 2012). Again, much of what we know comes from investigations of helping that does not include SV or IPV. House et al. (2013) examined the development of cooperation and helping behavior across a number of countries. Interestingly, they found similarity in helping and cooperation in early childhood across cultures. Differences then began to emerge and grow through middle childhood and into adulthood, suggesting to the authors the importance of cultural socialization in creating differences particularly in helping that carried potential costs. This is consistent with discussions of moral courage, helping that carries potential costs to the bystander, which is described as influenced by social and political contexts that impact the access to power and support a particular bystander may have (Osswald et al. 2010).

Communities in cultures that place more emphasis on the well-being of the group versus the individual are associated with greater helping in some studies (Levine et al. 2001) but such in-group focus also seems to inhibit helping strangers (Knafo 2009). In relation to SV and IPV, one recent study suggests that stronger ethnic identity was related to greater intent to help in SV and IPV situations at least among college students (Lee 2014). Other studies found that race and culture may impact correlates of bystander action as well. In relation to bullying, while the level of bystander action was similar in two different countries, the correlates (who, where, when) were different between Italy and Singapore (Pozzoli et al. 2012) and types of helping were different between Estonian and Russian-Estonian teenagers (Tamm and Tulvost 2015). Among a sample of U.S. college students, Black students engaged in more bystander behaviors to address SV and these behaviors were more influenced by supportive bystander peer norms than White students (Brown et al. 2014). This shows that bystander opportunities and challenges may be framed by culture in many different ways that we do not yet fully understand but that have implications for adapting our prevention strategies so that they are more culturally competent.

3.5.1.1 Online Versus in Person

Increasingly aspects of SV and IPV are extending into the online environment and thus so is potential bystander action (Bastiaensens et al. 2014). Research in this area has focused mainly on victimization and perpetration in online environments, suggesting that this is an area where bystander action could be helpful. Another line of research has focused on using electronic media to promote helping, through online bystander trainings for college students (e.g. Kleinsasser et al. 2015; Salazar et al. 2014) or through research that showed how prosocial video games or music increased helping by getting people thinking about things like helping and empathy and having those processes more front and center in their thinking (Greitemeyer 2011; Greitemeyer and Osswald 2010). However, bystanders are also active online and can choose to take action there. One study documented a variety of strategies students used online to confront bullying and harassment including telling the bully to stop, offering comfort to the victim, and trying to change the topic (Freis and Gurung 2013). Research also shows that some of the similar barriers to action exist online including that large social networks can easily create diffusion of responsibility (Blair et al. 2005; Martin and North 2015). While online resources for bystander education are proliferating, more research is needed about how to help bystanders take action using a range of social media and online environments.

3.5.1.2 Moving from Reactive to Proactive: A Different Setting for Bystander Action

Most of the settings where bystanders act involve an instance of SV or IPV. Yet another "when" of bystander response is proactive intervention when there is no risk at all. This involves getting more information, pursuing education, volunteering to raise awareness about sexual and relationship violence, displaying a logo or slogan that promotes violence prevention messages, starting conversations with friends and family about anti-violence messages, writing a letter to the editor to comment on a media story, encouraging community leaders to talk about SV and IPV, or working to enact new policies or laws that work against sexual violence and relationship abuse. Rogers (2002) diffusion of innovation theory reminds us that "innovators and early adopters", the first 15 % of a population to adopt new ideas or behaviors, have a powerful influence on the remainder of the community. Though much prevention and intervention work in the SV and IPV field relies on peer educators and community volunteers who help crisis center staff answer hotlines, plan events, and teach prevention messages in schools we know llittle about the effectiveness of such efforts and how to enhance actions that go beyond only reacting to risk in the moment (Anderson and Whiston 2005). Among college students this is when bystanders are least likely to get involved if given the opportunity (McMahon et al. 2015). A literature in social psychology on volunteerism, or the more public, scripted, planned type of helping that happens over time finds individuals with higher social capital, who have social or organizational support for their work and feel satisfied with the roles and work available to them are more likely to sustain this type of action (Amato 1990; Penner et al. 2005). If part of prevention work is getting more community members involved in prevention and intervention efforts, we need more research to better understand what may motivate them to do so. For example, several studies looked at men's involvement in SV and IPV prevention and what motivated them to become engaged (Barone et al. 2007; Casey and Ohler 2012; DeKeseredy et al. 2000). What is more, such bystanders have the potential to harness the power of social media to mobilize others to take action (Baek 2015 for research on use of social media to influence political mobilization and voting as an example).

3.6 Summary

- Factors that influence bystander action include aspects of the self that may form early in life and characteristics of the more immediate situation.
- A variety of factors across the social ecology help explain when individuals will act or not.
- Common themes across types of helping include: perceived efficacy, sense of responsibility, awareness of a problem, emotional arousal.
- Examining research specifically on bystanders related to SV and IPV also reveals new factors that are either unique to these problems or have not yet been studied in terms of bystander action more generally such as peer norms, relationship to people involved in the situation, and victim blaming attitudes.
- Prevention strategies need to teach flexibility to equip bystanders to manage the complex set of variables at play in any one situation.

3.7 Implications for Practice

Research on bystander action to date provides a number of lessons for prevention, In particular, prevention tools should focus on all of the correlates that research commonly shows help increase bystander action. Prevention tools should promote awareness. They need to build knowledge about what sexual and relationship violence are. Underlying this knowledge is also providing information about consent—what it is and how to actively seek and receive it (Borges et al. 2008). People need to feel responsible and a key piece of this is helping people see that the problems of sexual and relationship violence happen where they live. For example, what students said was most memorable about an educational program on one campus were the local community stories and statistics that made the problem relevant to their own particular experiences (Banyard et al. 2005).

Bystanders also need confidence to take action and be surrounded by others who model and support helping. The foundation for the particular actions that a bystander chooses come from developmental moments early in the lifespan—empathy, prosocial personality tendencies, moral development—that need to be the focus of prevention early on (Biglan et al. 2012). Cultivation of these seeds of helping will affect a variety of bystander actions, not just those for SV and IPV. Bystander action is also motivated by aspects of the current situation and broader community contexts that require prevention efforts at the level of the community to modify aspects of these situations. Bystander focused prevention should have at its core, activities that attend to the variables that appear most consistently in the literature including boosting confidence, increasing awareness, and building skills specific to SV and IPV situations. Prevention strategies need to be built on logic models and strategic plans that take into account the variety of factors across the social-ecological model that impact bystander action.

References

Ahrens, C. E., & Campbell, R. C. (2000). Assisting rape victims as they recover from rape. *The Impact on Friends Journal of Interpersonal Violence, 15*, 959–986.

Amato, P. R. (1990). Personality and social network involvement as predictors of helping behavior in everyday life. *Social Psychology Quarterly, 53*, 31–43.

Anderson, L. A., & Whiston, S. C. (2005). Sexual assault education programs: A meta-analytic examination of their effectiveness. *Psychology of Women Quarterly, 29*, 374–388.

Baek, Y. M. (2015). Political mobilization through social networking sites: The mobilizing power of political messaging received from SNS friends. *Computers in Human Behavior, 44*, 12–19.

Baldry, A. C., & Pagliaro, S. (2014). Helping victims of intimate partner violence: The influence of group norms among lay people and the police. *Psychology of Violence, 4*, 334–347.

Banyard, V. L. (2011). Who will help prevent sexual violence: Creating an ecological model of bystander intervention. *Psychology of Violence, 1*, 216–229.

Banyard, V. L., & Moynihan, M. M. (2011). Variation in bystander behavior related to sexual and intimate partner violence prevention: Correlates in a sample of college students. *Psychology of Violence, 1*, 287–301.

Banyard, V. L., Moynihan, M. M., & Plante, E. G. (2005). Rape prevention through bystander education: Bringing a broader community approach to sexual violence prevention. Final report for grant 2002-WG-BX-0009. National Institute of Justice. Accessed from https://www.ncjrs.gov/pdffiles1/nij/grants/208701.pdf.

Banyard, V. L., Moynihan, M. M., & Plante, E. G. (2007). Sexual violence prevention through bystander education: An experimental evaluation. *Journal of Community Psychology, 35*, 463–481.

Banyard, V. L., Eckstein, R., & Moynihan, M. M. (2010). Sexual violence prevention: The role of stages of change. *Journal of Interpersonal Violence, 25*, 111–135.

Banyard, V. L., Moynihan, M. M., Cares, A. C., & Warner, R. (2014). How do we know if it works? Measuring outcomes in bystander-focused abuse prevention on campuses. *Psychology of Violence, 4*, 101–115.

Banyard, V. L., Moynihan, M. M., Walsh, W., Cohn, E. S., & Ward, S. K. (2011). Friends of survivors: The community impact of unwanted sexual experiences. *Journal of Interpersonal Violence, 26*, 242–256.

Banyard, V., Weber, M., Grych, J., & Hamby, S. (in press). Where are the helpful bystanders? Ecological Niche and Victims' perceptions of bystander intervention. *Journal of Community Psychology*.

Barone, R. P., Wolgemuth, J. R., & Linder, C. (2007). Preventing sexual assault through engaging college men. *Journal of College Student Development, 48*, 585–594.

Bastiaensens, S., Vandebosch, H., Poels, K., Cleemput, K. V., DeSmet, A., & De Bourdeaudhuij, I. (2014). Cyberbulling on social network sites. An experimental study into bystanders' behavioral intentions to help the victim or reinforce the bully. *Computers in Human Behavior, 31*, 259–271.

Beeble, M. L., Post, L. A., Bybee, D., & Sullivan, C. M. (2008). Factors related to willingness to help survivors of intimate partner violence. *Journal of Interpersonal Violence, 23*, 1713–1729.

Bennett, S., & Banyard, V. (2014). Do friends really help friends? The effect of relational factors and perceived severity on bystander perception of sexual violence. Online first.

Bennett, S., Banyard, V. L., & Garnhart, L. (2014). To act or not to act, that is the question? Barriers and facilitators of bystander intervention. *Journal of Interpersonal Violence, 29*, 476–496.

Bennett, S., Banyard, V., & Edwards, K. (2015). The impact of the bystander's relationship with the victim and the perpetrator on intent to help in situations involving sexual violence. *Journal of Interpersonal Violence*.

Berkowitz, A. (2009). *Response ability: A complete guide on bystander behavior*. Chicago, IL: Beck and Co.

Bieneck, S., & Krahe, B. (2011). Blaming the victim and exonerating the perpetrator in cases of rape and robbery: Is there a double standard. *Journal of Interpersonal Violence, 26*, 1785–1797.

Biglan, A., Flay, B. R., Embry, D. D., & Sandler, I. N. (2012). The critical role of nurturing environments for promoting human well-being. *American Psychologist, 67*, 257–271.

Blair, C. A., Thompson, L. F., & Wuensc, K. L. (2005). Electronic helping behavior: the virtual presence of others makes a difference. *Basic and Applied Social Psychology, 27*, 171–178.

Borges, A., Banyard, V. L., & Moynihan, M. M. (2008). Clarifying consent: Primary prevention of sexual assault on a college campus. *Journal of Prevention and Intervention in the Community, 36*, 75–88.

Bronfenbrenner, U. (1977). Toward and experimental ecology of human development. *American Psychologist, 32*, 513–531.

Brown, A., Banyard, V. L., & Moynihan, M. M. (in press). The impact of perceived peer norms and gender, age, and race on bystander intentions and behaviors related to sexual violence. *Psychology of Women Quarterly*.

Burn, S. M. (2009). A situational model of sexual assault prevention through bystander intervention. *Sex Roles, 60*, 779–792.

Campbell, R., Sefl, T., Barnes, H. E., Ahrens, C. E., Wasco, S. M., & Zaragoza-Diesfeld, Y. (1999). Community services for rape survivors: Enhancing psychological well-being or increasing trauma? *Journal of Consulting and Clinical Psychology, 67*, 847–858.

Caravita, S. C. S., Gini, G., & Pozzoli, T. (2012). Main and moderated effects of moral cognition and status on bullying and defending. *Aggressive Behavior, 38*, 456–468.

Cares, A. C., Banyard, V. L., Moynihan, M. M., Williams, L. M., Potter, S. J., & Stapleton, J. G. (2015). Changing attitudes about being a bystander to violence: translating an in-person education program to a new campus. *Violence Against Women, 21*, 165–187.

Carlo, G., & Randall, B. A. (2002). The development of a measure of prosocial behaviors for late adolescents. *Journal of Youth and Adolescence, 31*, 31–44.

Carlo, G., Fabes, R. A., Laible, D., & Kupanoff, K. (1999). Early adolescence and prosocial/moral behavior II: The role of social and contextual influences. *Journal of Early Adolescence, 19*, 133–147.

Carlo, G., Hausmann, A., Christiansen, S., & Randall, B. A. (2003). Sociocognitive and behavioral correlates of a measure of prosocial tendencies for adolescents. *Journal of Early Adolescence, 23*, 107–134.

Carlson, M. (2008). I'd rather go along and be considered a man: Masculinity and bystander intervention. *Journal of Men's Studies, 16*, 3–17.

Casey, E. A., & Ohler, K. (2012). Being a positive bystander: Male antiviolence allies' experiences of "stepping up". *Journal of Interpersonal Violence, 27*, 62–83.

Chabot, H. F., Tracy, T. L., Manning, C. A., & Poisson, C. A. (2009). Sex, attribution, and severity influence intervention decisions of informal helpers in domestic violence. *Journal of Interpersonal Violence, 24*, 1696–1713.

Chaurand, N., & Brauer, M. (2008). What determines social control? People's reactions to counternormative behaviors in urban environment. *Journal of Applied Social Psychology, 38*, 1689–1715.

References

Christy, C. A., & Voigt, H. (1994). Bystander responses to public episodes of child abuse. *Journal of Applied Social Psychology, 24,* 824–847.

Coke, C. D., Batson, J. S., & McDavis, K. (1978). Empathic mediation of helping: A two-stage model. *Journal of Personality and Social Psychology, 36,* 752–766.

DeKeseredy, W. S., Schwartz, M. D., & Alvi, S. (2000). The role of profeminist men in dealing with woman abuse on the Canadian College Campus. *Violence Against Women, 6,* 918–935.

Dovidio, J. F., Piliavin, J. A., Gaertner, S. L., Schroeder, D. A., & Clark, R. D. (1991). The arousal: Cost-reward model and the process of intervention: A review of the evidence. *Prosocial behavior: Review of Personality and Social Psychology, 12,* 86–118.

Dovidio, J., Piliavin, J. A., Schroeder, D., & Penner, L. (2006). *The social psychology of prosocial behavior.* Mahwah, NJ: Erlbaum.

Durlak, J. A., Weissberg, R. P., Dymnicki, A. B., Taylor, R. D., & Schellinger, K. B. (2011). The impact of enhancing students' social and emotional learning: A meta-analysis of school-based universal interventions. *Child Development, 82,* 405–432.

Eagley, A. H., & Crowley, M. (1986). Gender and helping behavior: A meta-analytic review of the social psychological literature. *Psychological Bulletin, 100,* 283–308.

Eagly, A. H. (2009). The his and hers of prosocial behavior: an examination of the social psychology of gender. *American Psychologist, 64,* 644–658.

Edwards, K. M., Dardis, C. M., & Gidycz, C. A. (2012). Women's disclosure of dating violence: A mixed methodological study. *Feminism and Psychology, 22,* 507–517.

Edwards, K. M., Mattingly, M. J., Dixon, K. J., & Banyard, V. L. (2014). Community matters: intimate partner violence among rural young adults. *American Journal of Community Psychology, 53,* 198–207.

Eisenberg, N., Guthrie, I. K., Murphy, B. C., Shepard, S. A., Cumberland, A., & Carlo, G. (1999). Consistency and development of prosocial dispositions: A longitudinal study. *Child Development, 70,* 1360–1372.

Eisenberg, N., Guthrie, I. K., Cumberland, A., Murphy, B. C., Shepard, S. A., Zhou, Q., & Carlo, G. (2002). Prosocial development in early adulthood: A longitudinal study. *Journal of Personality and Social Psychology, 82,* 993–1006.

Fabiano, P. M., Perkins, H. W., Berkowitz, A., Linkenbach, J., & Stark, C. (2003). Engaging men as social justice allies in ending violence against women: Evidence for a social norms approach. *Journal of American College Health, 52,* 105–112.

Ferrans, S. D., Selman, R. L., & Feigenberg, L. F. (2012). Rules of the culture and personal needs: Witnesses' decision-making processes to deal with situations of bullying in middle school. *Harvard Educational Review, 82,* 445–470.

Finkelor, D., Vanderminden, J., Turner, H., Shattuck, A., & Hamby, S. (2014). Youth exposure to violence prevention programs in a national sample. *Child Abuse and Neglect, 38,* 677–686.

Fischer, P., Greitemeyer, T., Pollozek, F., & Frey, D. (2006). The unresponsive bystander: Are bystanders more responsive in dangerous emergencies? *European Journal of Social Psychology, 36,* 267–278.

Fischer, P., Krueger, J. I., Greitemeyer, T., Vogrincic, C., Kastenmuller, A., & Frey, D. (2011). The bystander-effect: A meta-analytic review on bystander intervention in dangerous and non-dangerous emergencies. *Psychological Bulletin, 132,* 517–537.

Flay, B. R., Snyder, F. J., & Petraitis, J. (2009). The theory of triadic influence. In R. J. DiClemente, R. A. Crosby, & M. C. Kegler (Eds.), *Emerging theories in health promotion practice and research* (2nd ed., pp. 452–510). San Francisco, CA: Jossey-Bass.

Fledderjohann, J., & Johnson, D. R. (2012). What predicts the actions taken toward observed child neglect? The influence of community context and bystander characteristics. *Social Science Quarterly, 93,* 1030–1052.

Frazier, P., Greer, C., Gabrielsen, S., Tennen, H., Park, C., & Tomich, P. (2013). The relation between trauma exposure and prosocial behavior. *Psychological Trauma: Theory, Research, Practice, and Policy, 5,* 286–294.

Freis, S. D., & Gurung, R. A. R. (2013). A facebook analysis of helping behavior in online bullying. *Psychology of Popular Media Culture, 2*, 11–19.

Fry, D. A., Messinger, A. M., Rickert, V. I., O'Connor, M. K., Palmetto, N., Lessel, H., & Davidson, L. L. (2013). Adolescent relationship violence: Help-seeking and help-giving behaviors among peers. *Journal of Urban Health: Bulletin of the New York Academy of Medicine.*

Frye, V. (2007). The informal social control of intimate partner violence against women: Exploring personal attitudes and perceived neighborhood social cohesion. *Journal of Community Psychology, 35*, 1001–1018.

Frye, V., et al. (2012). Informal social control of intimate partner violence against women: Results from a concept mapping study of urban neighborhoods. *Journal of Community Psychology, 40*, 828–844.

George, D., Carroll, P., Kersnick, R., & Calderon, K. (1998). Gender-related patterns of helping among friends. *Psychology of Women Quarterly, 22*, 685–704.

Gracia, E., & Herrero, J. (2006). Public attitudes toward reporting partner violence against women and reporting behavior. *Journal of Marriage and Family, 68*, 759–768.

Gracia, E., Garcia, F., & Lila, M. (2009). Public responses to intimate partner violence against women: The influence of perceived severity and personal responsibility. *The Spanish Journal of Psychology, 12*, 648–656.

GreenDot, Etc. (2015). An overview of the Green Dot strategy. Accessed from http://www.calcasa.org/wp-content/uploads/2011/04/Curriculum-Summary.pdf. March 4, 2015.

Greitemeyer, T. (2011). Effects of prosocial media on prosocial behavior: when and why does media exposure affect helping and aggression? *Current Directions in Psychological Science, 20*, 251–255.

Greitemeyer, T., & Osswald, S. (2010). Effects of prosocial video games on prosocial behavior. *Journal of Personality and Social Psychology, 98*, 211–221.

Greitemeyer, T., Fischer, P., Kastenmuller, A., & Frey, D. (2006). Civil courage and helping behavior: Differences and similarities. *European Psychologist, 11*, 90–98.

Greitemeyer, T., Osswald, S., Fischer, P., & Frey, D. (2007). Civil courage: Implicit theories, related concepts, and measurement. *The Journal of Positive Psychology, 2*, 115–119.

Hamby, S., Weber, M., Grych, J. & Banyard, V. (2015). What difference do bystanders make? The association of victim outcomes with bystander involvement in a community sample. *Psychology of Violence.*

Hektner, J. M., & Swenson, C. A. (2012). Links from teacher beliefs to peer victimization and bystander intervention: Tests of mediating processes. *Journal of Early Adolescence, 32*, 516–536.

House, B. R., Silk, J. B., Henrich, J., Barrett, H. C., Scelza, B. A., Boyette, A. H., et al. (2013). Ontogeny of prosocial behavior across diverse societies. *Proceedings of the National Academy of Sciences of the United States of America, 10*, 14586–14591.

Katz, J., Pazienza, R., Olin, R., & Rich, H. (2014). That's what friends are for: Bystander responses to friends or strangers at risk for party rape victimization. *Journal of Interpersonal Violence.* Online first publication.

Kelly, J. A. (2004). Popular opinion leaders and HIV prevention peer education: resolving discrepant findings, and implications for the development of effective community programmes. *AIDS CARE, 16*, 139–150.

Kleinsasser, A., Jouriles, E. N., McDonald, R., & Rosenfield, D. (2015). An online bystander intervention program for the prevention of sexual violence. *Psychology of Violence, 5*(3), 227–235.

Knafo, A., Schwartz, S. A., & Levine, R. V. (2009). Helping strangers is lower in embedded cultures. *Journal of Cross-Cultural Psychology, 40*, 875–879.

Lamy, L., Fischer-Lokou, J., & Gueguen, N. (2012). Priming emotion concepts and helping behavior: How unlived emotions can influence action. *Social Behavior and Personality, 40*, 55–62.

References

Laner, M. R., Benin, M. H., & Ventrone, N. A. (2001). Bystander attitudes toward victims of violence: Who's worth helping? *Deviant Behavior, 22*, 23–42.

Latané, B., & Darley, J. M. (1970). *The unresponsive bystander: Why doesn't he help?* New York, NY: Appleton-Century-Crofts.

Latané, B., & Nida, S. (1981). Ten years of research on group size and helping. *Psychological Bulletin, 89*, 308–324.

Latta, R. E., & Goodman, L. A. (2011). Intervening in partner violence against women: A grounded theory exploration of informal network members' experiences. *The Counseling Psychologist, 39*, 973–1023.

Lazarus, K., & Signal, T. (2013). Who will help in situations of intimate partner violence: Exploring personal attitudes and bystander behaviours. *International Journal of Criminology and Sociology, 2*, 199–209.

Lee, E. T. (2014). *The relationship between cultural and psychological factors and their effects on bystander interventions in sexual intimate partner violence (IPV) situations.* Unpublished master's thesis, California State University, Sacramento.

Leone, R. M., Parrott, D. J., Swartout, K. M., & Tharp, A. D. (2015). *Masculinity and bystander attitudes: Moderating effects of masculine gender role stress.* Online first: Psychology of Violence.

Levine, M., & Crowther, S. (2008). The responsive bystander: How social group membership and group size can encourage as well as inhibit bystander intervention. *Journal of Personality and Social Psychology, 95*, 1429–1439.

Levine, R. V., Norenzayan, A., & Philbrick, K. (2001). Cross-cultural differences in helping strangers. *Journal of Cross-Cultural Psychology, 32*, 543–560.

Levine, M., Prosser, A., Evans, D., & Reicher, S. (2005). Identity and emergency interventions: How social group membership and inclusiveness of group boundaries shape helping behavior. *Personality and Social Psychology Bulletin, 31*, 443–453.

Levine, M., Taylor, P. J., & Best, R. (2011). Third parties, violence, and conflict resolution: The role of group size and collective action in the microregulation of violence. *Psychological Science, 22*, 406–412.

Levine, M., Lowe, R., Best, R., & Heim, D. (2012). "We police it ourselves:" Group processes in the escalation and regulation of violence in the night-time economy. *European Journal of Social Psychology, 42*, 924–932.

Martin, K. K., & North, A. C. (2015). Diffusion of responsibility on social network sites. *Computers in Human Behavior, 44*, 124–131.

McMahon, S. (2010). Rape myth beliefs and bystander attitudes among incoming college students. *Journal of American College Health, 59*, 3–11.

McMahon, S., Banyard, V., & McMahon, S. (2015). Incoming college students' bystander behaviors to prevent sexual violence. *Journal of College Student Development, 56*, 488–493.

McMahon, S., Banyard, V., Palmer, J. E., Murphy, M.J., & Gidycz, C. A. (in press) (b). Chances to reduce sexual violence: Measuring bystander behavior in the context of opportunity to help. *Journal of Interpersonal Violence*.

Mollen, S., Rimalc, R. N., Ruitera, R. A. C., Jangd, S. A., & Koka, G. (2013). Intervening or interfering? The influence of injunctive and descriptive norms on intervention behaviours in alcohol consumption contexts. *Psychology and Health, 28*, 561–578.

Nicksa, S. C. (2010). *College bystanders' predicted reactions to witnessing sexual assault: The impact of gender, community, bystander experience, and relationship to the victim.* Unpublished doctoral dissertation, Northeastern University, Boston, MA.

Nicksa, S. C. (2014). Bystander's willingness to report theft, physical assault, and sexual assault: The impact of gender, anonymity, and relationship with the offender. *Journal of Interpersonal Violence, 29*, 217–236.

Osswald, S., Greitemeyer, T., Fischer, P., & Frey, D. (2010). What is moral courage? Definition, explication, and classification of a complex construct. In C. L. Purry & S. J. Lopez (Eds.), *The psychology of courage: modern research on an ancient virtue.* Washington, D.C.: American Psychological Association.

Parrott, D. J., Tharp, A. T., Swartout, K. M., Miller, C. A., Hall, G. C. N., & George, W. H. (2012). Validity for an integrated laboratory analogue of sexual aggression and bystander intervention. *Aggressive Behavior, 38*, 309–321.

Paternotte, C. (2011). Rational choice theory. In I. C. Jarvie & J. Zamora-Bonilla (Eds.), *The SAGE handbook of the philosophy of social sciences*, pp. 307–321.

Paul, L. A., & Gray, M. J. (2011). Sexual assault programming on college campuses: Using social psychological belief and behavior change principles to improve outcomes. *Trauma Violence Abuse, 12*, 99–109.

Penner, L. A., Dovidio, J. F., Piliavin, J. A., & Schroeder, D. A. (2005). Prosocial behavior: Multilevel perspectives. *Annual Review of Psychology, 56*, 365–392.

Pinchevsky, G. M., & Wright, E. M. (2012). The impact of neighborhoods on intimate partner violence and victimization. *Trauma, Violence, and Abuse, 13*(2), 112–132.

Planty, M. (2002). *Third-party involvement in violent crime, 1993–1999*. Bureau of Justice Statistics Special Report. Washington, D.C.: U.S. Department of Justice. NCJ189100.

Potter, S. J., & Stapleton, J. G. (2012). Translating sexual assault prevention from a college campus to a United States military installation: piloting the know-your-power bystander social marketing campaign. *Journal of Interpersonal Violence, 27*, 1593–1621.

Pozzoli, T., & Gini, G. (2010). Active defending and passive bystanding behavior in bullying: The role of personal characteristics and perceived peer pressure. *Journal of Abnormal Child Psychology, 38*, 815–827.

Pozzoli, T., Ang, R. P., & Gini, G. (2012a). Bystanders' reactions to bullying: A cross-cultural analysis of personal correlates among Italian and Singaporean students. *Social Development, 21*, 686–703.

Pozzoli, T., Gini, G., & Vieno, A. (2012b). The role of individual correlates and class norms in defending and passive bystanding behavior in bullying: A multilevel analysis. *Child Development, 83*, 1917–1931.

Rogers, E. M. (2002). Diffusion of preventive innovations. *Addictive Behaviors, 27*, 989–993.

Rothman, E. F., Johnson, R. M., Young, R., Weinberg, J., Azrael, D., & Molnar, B. E. (2011). Neighborhood-level factors associated with physical dating violence perpetration: Results of a representative survey conducted in Boston, MA. *Journal of Urban Health: Bulletin of the New York Academy of Medicine, 88*, 201–213.

Ruggieria, S., Friemelb, T., Sticcac, F., Perrenc, S., & Alsaker, F. (2013). Selection and influence effects in defending a victim of bullying: The moderating effects of school context. *Procedia—Social and Behavioral Sciences, 79*, 117–126.

Rushton, J. P. (1978). Urban density and altruism: Helping strangers in a Canadian city, suburb, and small town. *Psychological Reports, 43*, 987–990.

Salazar, L. F., Vivolo-Kantor, A., Hardin, J., & Berkowitz, A. (2014). A web-based sexual violence bystander intervention for male college students: Randomized control trial. *Journal of Medical Internet Research*, 16, e203.

Sapouna, M. (2010). Collective efficacy in the school context: Does it help explain bullying and victimization among Greek primary and secondary school students? *Journal of Interpersonal Violence, 25*, 1912–1927.

Shotland, R. L., & Straw, M. K. (1976). Bystander response to an assault: When a man attacks a woman. *Journal of Personality and Social Psychology, 34*, 990–999.

Slater, M., Rovira, A, Southern, R., Swapp, D., Zhang, J. J., Campbell, C. & Levine, M. (2013). Bystander responses to a violent incident in an immersive virtual environment. *PLOS ONE 8*, e52766.

Stein, J. L. (2007). Peer educators and close friends as predictors of male college students' willingness to prevent rape. *Journal of College Student Development, 48*, 75–89.

Suarez, E., & Gadalla, T. M. (2010). Stop blaming the victim: A meta-analysis of rape myths. *Journal of Interpersonal Violence, 25*, 2010–2035.

Tamm, A., & Tulviste, T. (2015). The role of gender, values, and culture in adolescent bystanders' strategies. *Journal of Interpersonal Violence, 30*, 382–399.

Ullman, S. (2010). *Talking about sexual assault: Society's response to survivors*. Washington, DC: American Psychological Association.

Veenstra, R., Lindenberg, S., Huitsing, G., Sainio, M., & Salmivalli, C. (2014). The role of teachers in bullying: The relation between antibullying attitudes, efficacy, and efforts to reduce bullying. *Journal of Educational Psychology, 106*, 1135–1143.

West, A., & Wandrei, M. L. (2002). Intimate partner violence: A model for predicting interventions by informal helpers. *Journal of Interpersonal Violence, 17*, 972–986.

White House Task Force to Protect Students from Sexual Assault (2014). Notalone.gov.

White, C. H., & Malkowski, J. (2014). Communicative challenges of bystander intervention: Impact of goals and message design logic on strategies college students use to intervene in drinking situations. *Health Communication, 29*, 93–104.

Zimbardo, P. G., & Leippe, M. R. (1991). *The psychology of attitude change and social influence*. New York: McGraw Hill.

Zhong, L. Y. (2010). Bystander intervention and fear of crime: Evidence from two chinese communities. *International Journal of Offender Therapy and Comparative Criminology, 54*, 250–263.

Chapter 4
Bystander Action Coils: Moving Beyond the Situational Model

> *That was my first encounter with [sexual assault] and I felt like a terrible person and I didn't umm I don't know I just didn't know how to handle the situation...*
> —College student describing being a bystander to an instance of sexual violence

Abstract Research on bystander action often looks at different discrete variables that might hinder or promote stepping up to help someone in danger. How then do we assemble these pieces into a broader model that explains bystander behavior? This Chapter begins with the most well-known model of bystander intervention, the Situational Model of Latané and Darley and explores other frameworks developed since then. These broader models have limitations for understanding the unique context of interpersonal violence, especially sexual and relationship violence. Thus, the chapter builds a revised model of bystander action—Bystander Action Coils. This framework pays attention to developing new helping scripts in situations of interpersonal violence, attending to the relational context of bystander action in these circumstances, looks at broader community and cultural factors that may influence bystander behavior, and highlights the importance of understanding more about the consequences of different bystander actions. Details of this revised model are described.

Keywords Bystander action · Process model · Community · Development

The previous chapter reviewed what we currently know about bystander action as a basis for our prevention efforts. What we learn is that there are a number of key variables that can be leveraged to promote helpful bystander action across the continuum of sexual and relationship violence. To learn about the conditions for mobilizing helpful bystanders I drew from three different literatures that span a number of disciplines: research on general helping and low cost helping in clearly defined emergencies like assisting someone who has dropped something, helping someone with a task like crossing the street, helping someone with a broken down vehicle or a medical problem; research on situations requiring "moral courage" (Osswald et al. 2010)—more dangerous situations that carry high potential negative costs for bystanders; and finally the growing research specific to bystanders to SV and IPV. What we learned is that there are many common factors for activating bystanders across these situations—efficacy or confidence to act, awareness of the problem, a sense of responsibility to act. Research on SV and IPV more specifically also highlighted new factors that need to be attended to including peer and community norms, attitudes related specifically to violence including victim blame, community collective efficacy and the importance of behaviors and attitudes modeled by community leaders. What we also learned was that most of the research looked at different pieces of the puzzle in a rather disconnected manner. One study may focus on the presence or absence of other bystanders but not look at how that is also connected to variables like awareness or confidence. Effective prevention work that aims to build bystander action requires that we connect the dots in a roadmap that can help us highlight better how these different pieces or correlates fit together.

4.1 MODELS—Pulling Individual Variables Together

Several theorists in the area of bystander intervention connect variables across the who, what, when, why, and where (Dovidio et al. 1991; Latané and Darley 1970), focusing in particular on the proximal building blocks for bystanders in the immediate situation. These are things we can actually influence rather than more distal factors that may be harder to change. This is important for prevention work. The most well-known of these is the situational model of Latané and Darley and this theory forms the basis of much bystander focused prevention to date. Their model does not seek to explain nuances of how a bystander will take action or how this may differ by situation. Rather it seems to outline a more universal template for taking action or not. First, a bystander must notice the situation and label someone as needing help. The bystander must then feel a personal sense of responsibility for doing something about the situation and have the skills to act. At each place in the model, the variables summarized in the previous chapter can help tip the balance toward or away from action.

A second general model of helping is the arousal cost reward model (Dovidio et al. 1991). What this model highlights is that distress in another person causes unpleasant feelings in observers that bystanders are motivated to reduce. Bystanders seek to do this through actions that will most effectively address the situation with the fewest personal costs. This model integrates the "why" with "when" of helping but also suggests that variability in individual characteristics, the "who," such as empathy will also be important to the model.

What is important to note is that the situational model is built mostly on helping strangers and discrete, one time incidents that present few potential social costs to bystanders. Models of moral courage provide an alternate view that take into account important issues like negative consequences for bystanders

(Osswald et al. 2010). Moral courage is a model that describes helping when an injustice is conftonted (such as defending someone being discriminated against or degraded, treated unfairly because of a minority status, or whistleblowing about unfair or unethical practices). A key feature of moral courage is that active bystanders face negative consequences, face offenders who are threatening, and bystanders are acting for a greater social good. Moral courage has a different set of correlates than more general helping actions according to research (Osswald et al. 2010). For example, the classic bystander effect of diffusion of responsibility was not found for instances of moral courage. Situations of moral courage triggered heightened awareness and greater emotional arousal than general helping. Positive mood enhances helping but moral courage is enhanced instead by anger, sense of justice, and the presence of strong social norms and examples of others modeling morally courageous acts (see Osswald et al. 2010 for a review). Below I discuss how these foundational theories present limitations for understanding bystander action in the context of SV and IPV.

4.2 Limits of Models for Understanding Sexual and Relationship Violence

The uniqueness and complexity of sexual and relationship violence presents challenges to the bystander models summarized above. Indeed, Pozzoli and Gini (2010) described how taking action to help victims of bullying differed from more general prosocial helping behavior. They state, "Intervening in favor of the victim in the context of peer aggression represents a risky behavior, since the helper confronts a powerful bully and, sometimes, even his/her supporters. Given the particular conditions in which it occurs, intervention in favor of the victim of bullying should be regarded as a complex behavior that include not only the positive perception of the victim, but also a 'moral' assumption of personal responsibility to intervene from the defender (p. 816)". Indeed, each component of the situational model has limitations for understanding helping in this unique and complicated context, a point Osswald et al. (2010) made when calling for new models of behaviors they describe as moral courage. The situational model, since it is the most often cited, is used below to illustrate these limitations in more detail.

The first aspect of the model is to notice and label the situation as a problem. Research is clear that more obvious and collectively defined emergency situations produce more ready bystander actions (Fischer et al. 2011). Sexual and relationship violence, however, represent a continuum of behaviors (McMahon and Banyard 2012) not all of which are agreed upon as harmful. For example, many people do not see harassing comments or unwanted touching as serious but rather may define it as playful or flirtatious behavior. Indeed, popular opinion surveys show that people have a difficult time identifying what dating violence is, for example, and editorials, another indicator of community opinions, often call into question even instances of sexual assault (Chan 2007). This context of disagreement about what behaviors constitute sexual or relationship violence creates problems for bystanders being able to notice and accurately label what they see at the start of the helping process. It may cause doubt about whether intervention is needed. For example, the comments that followed a recent New York Times article about bystander intervention (Winerip 2014) and sexual assault revealed considerable disagreement about whether unwanted advances at a party or in a bar were a problem that should be addressed or part of normal young adult sexual behavior scripts. Scholars highlight both historical and ongoing debates about what consent to sexual activity is and when someone is too incapacitated to give consent (McGregor 2005). Sexual and relationship violence is also not one behavior—it is a continuum of risk factors. So we are asking people to become aware of a variety of things at the same time. These issues present hurdles for bystander awareness that are not a factor for other types of helping situations where bystander action has been explored. Indeed, this is one way that SV and IPV present challenges even for the model of moral courage, a model that highlights that situations that call for moral courage are easily and quickly identified.

Bystanders must not only be aware and label the situation as sexual or relationship violence but they must also feel responsible for taking action. Again, community norms can create confusion for bystanders. Flood and Pease (2009) described the persistence of rape myths. These are attitudes and beliefs about sexual assault. While these have most often been researched in relation to their impact on victims (reducing disclosure, increasing shame and self blame) and perpetrators (condoning their behaviors), these myths can also impact bystanders even beyond identification of the situation as noted above. For example, prevalent norms related to sexual and relationship violence are that it is a private matter or that victims are to blame for what happens given what they wear, what they are drinking, where they are walking, or their choice to remain in a relationship (Goodman and Epstein 2011). These notions of privacy encourage bystanders not to see themselves as responsible for helping as the belief is that couples should be left alone to work out their own problems. What is more, rape myths and belief systems may impact the type of arousal bystanders experience. What happens if they see a victim in distress but rather than taking action to help to decrease that arousal, they reframe the situation, blame the victim and thus determine the person is not deserving of assistance—an option that can be encouraged by community norms that support myths about interpersonal violence (Dovidio et al. 1991). In that instance emotional discomfort has been reduced but not through helping. Myths of false reports and of victim blame work against bystanders taking responsibility for stepping in.

Related to this issue of responsibility is the limitation that much of the research on the situational model is based on helping strangers rather than friends. This makes sense since this area of study began in the social psychology laboratory or in controlled field studies where a believable confederate who posed as needing help was required. This confederate needed to be someone the research participant did not know. In the case of sexual and relationship violence, however, much helping involves friends and as reviewed previously, the quality or helping process may look different for friends versus strangers. Certainly the motives for helping may differ if you are helping a friend versus a stranger, though this is a question that has not been explored in the research literature. Most motives for helping are based on having some sort of relationship with the person such that you expect you will receive something in return or feel related to the person in such a way that their well-being will impact your own well-being. It is less clear how such theories of motivation explain helping strangers.

Latané and Darley's model also explains one time helping where the end point is the bystander action. But when you look at narratives of people's experience of helping, particularly in cases of relationship abuse, they usually talked about friends and they often talked about a process of helping or a series of actions that unfolded over time (Latta and Goodman 2011). Friends and family described helping over time that included periods of getting involved and needing to pull back. In my own work I similarly found at times that college students described ongoing instances of bystander action in relation to helping friends who were dealing with sexual assault or relationship violence. This contrasted with more general examples of helping described by these same participants, who tended to describe those as instances of helping both friends and strangers with one time, fairly specific needs like borrowing homework, holding the door open, walking someone home from a party or lending class notes. This fits with work by Osswald et al. (2010) who documented differences in correlates of actions taken when there was a strong potential for negative consequences, critiquing models like the situational model for focusing on situations where there were lower potential intervention costs.

A final aspect of the situational model is evaluating one's skills to intervene. Part of this piece of the model is assessing the costs and benefits to helping. Again, the circumstances of sexual and relationship violence present unique hurdles for bystanders including the wide range of potential actions to be taken, perceptions of bystanders by others, bystanders' own confidence and skills as well as safety. As noted earlier, sexual and relationship abuse represent a continuum of behaviors. Thus, helping actions are numerous and can take many different forms from more indirect strategies (calling in professional helpers or trying to distract a person to get them out of the situation) to more direct (confronting perpetrators, trying to remove a victim from a situation). This stands in contrast to other types of helping situations (e.g. someone has a medical emergency so you call 911; someone drops their books so you help pick them up; someone's car has broken down so you offer to help change the tire) that present a more narrow range of potential helping solutions. How do we help bystanders to sexual and relationship violence expand their ideas for how to help and make choices from among these options that do not leave the bystander feeling overwhelmed?

Finally, some of the situations in which we want people to intervene are dangerous (Hamby et al. 2015; Janson and Hazler 2004). How do we consider safety beyond seeing it as a barrier to helping? For example, across forms of victimizations, victims reported that bystanders were most often hurt in situations of sexual violence (Hamby et al. 2015). I found that college students often cited an unwillingness to take action on campus in relation to party situations where underage drinking occurred. They expressed concern that they would be sanctioned for their own behavior like underage drinking, or the behavior of surrounding peers, if professional helpers (campus security, administrators, and resident assistants) were called in. As one student, "they can help without getting in trouble themselves. I think a lot of people are very willing to help if they don't see themselves getting in trouble in the outcome." Yet another student remarked, "We can't really help this kid 'cause we're drinking too," he said. "So we're all gonna get screwed."

The issue is that our current models for understanding helping are not complex enough to map the landscape of sexual and relationship violence that bystanders must navigate. We need a more integrated view that pulls pieces from these different models and puts them together to help us see all of the components we have to pay attention to in order to mobilize bystanders or defenders. We need to start to look at all of these in one place, blending ideas across often siloed topics. The result is a model that can help push our thinking about how all types of bystander action happen, though of current concern is how it better positions us to understand bystanders to SV and IPV. A new model will enable the design of more effective prevention strategies to mobilize them.

4.3 Aspects of SV and IPV Bystander Action that Need Attention in a Revised Model

When we review the more specific research on SV and IPV bystanders, there are three key lessons learned that have implications for a revised model. (1) We need to help individuals develop new helping scripts rather than just relying on previous learned and practiced impulses and strategies to help. (2) We need a more relational model of bystander action given that bystanders most likely know victims and perpetrators in the situations they witness. (3) We need to broaden our consideration of contextual factors, the ecological niche in which the bystander action takes place. Below I explain each of these lessons or challenges posed by SV and IPV action. I then present a model that will blend both elements of previous bystander action models with components that better address these new factors.

4.3.1 Challenging What Helping Means: The Need for New Scripts

Active bystanding to help victims of interpersonal violence carries much greater risks for the helper and involves a more complex set of variables that influence whether the situation will improve or worsen. Thus, an added complication for bystanders is that the usual cognitive scripts they use for pro-social behavior and helping may be of little use (Osswald et al. 2010). Researchers have described the importance of these "behavior social scripts" (Avery et al. 2009). They describe these as guidelines for how one should usually behave in different social situations and assert that some scripts are clearer or better-known than others. Being in situations without a good script can cause anxiety and concern about what to do as, "in

4.3 Aspects of SV and IPV Bystander Action ...

unscripted situations, there are fewer norms and cues available guiding individual choices regarding appropriate speech and behavior. This lack of situational signals renders common heuristics governing interpersonal interaction ineffective. The result is a high degree of uncertainty concerning what to say or do (Avery et al. 2009, p. 1389)." To date, however, questions such as these have not been discussed in relation to bystander action for SV and IPV and how prevention work needs to prepare individuals to handle this mismatch between how they usually help others and what the SV or IPV situation may require.

Recent qualitative studies (one on a college campus and one in a rural community) suggested that how individuals described how "helping" in general happens in a community and how helping in relation to SV and IPV happen were quite different (Edwards and Banyard 2014). For example, one college student described, "I wanted to step in and try to talk, but I didn't know what was going on or what was being discussed so I just didn't, because I didn't know my place in the situation." What is interesting is that in response to questions about helping in general, individuals described small kindnesses, giving someone directions or helping with homework, as well as more significant time investments in listening to a friend's problems or organizing a community fund raiser for someone with medical bills to pay. When asked about helping in situations of sexual or relationship violence, however, participants often said they were not sure how to help and were concerned about what was best to do or were concerned that helping related to relationship abuse made something private too public or that it might cause negative effects for those who try to help:

> That aspect of not wanting to get that public attention drawn into a negative situation, shining a bad light on the family. Everyone in town is known by everyone else, so a negative situation would also be known to everyone else....There's no education for the community to understand what to do in those situations.
>
> I think a lot of people don't help either I mean they just are afraid to get involved, they don't want to poke their noses into other people's business if they don't have to because they're afraid they'll get sucked into it as well. Because I mean if they get involved you know then they might possibly become victims of ridicule and rumors themselves.

They described trying to help more privately by helping friends find safety or by trying over time to figure out what the victim needed.

Such descriptions suggest that there may be a schema mismatch between how individuals think about helping more generally, and the helping situations they are confronted with regarding sexual and relationship abuse. Sources of this mismatch include that there are a number of helping strategies or options and that bystanders may often need to try a series of actions to end the risky situation. Indeed this is also the promise of knowing perpetrators and victims that bystander action may not just be a one shot opportunity to help but may provide opportunities to loop back and try again or try something different. Bystanders may get second or third chances to do or say something. Further, bystanders may need to try multiple strategies and likely make choices based on the goals they have for trying to influence a situation, what have been termed "different communicative intervention strategies (p. 95)" (White and Malkowski 2014). The prevention curriculum designed by GreenDot, Etc. describes the "3 D's of bystander intervention" as "Direct, Distract, and Delegate"

(GreenDot, Etc. 2015) and to which I would add, "distance." These categories describe the variety of ways that bystanders can choose to act—by confronting perpetrators, approaching victims, creating distractions that diffuse the situation, getting others to help, or finding ways to remove the potential perpetrator or victim from the situation. This is a greater set of choices then the array of possible actions for helping someone across the street or assisting someone with a medical emergency and thus will require more complex and flexible helping scripts.

Beyond types of actions, bystanders can also take on a variety of roles in relation to SV and IPV, what we might call action roles. This not really been discussed in the bystander literature. Research on bullying uses the term "defenders" to separate bystanders who step in on behalf of victims rather than those who may join in the bullying (Pozzoli and Gini 2013). This defender role seems to capture well the series of actions described in the paragraph above. They are the people who are in the midst of the at-risk situation. As discussed, earlier, however, there are other situations where bystanders are needed and other roles they can play. For example, "supporters" are those bystanders who receive disclosures from victims and are in a position to promote recovery or increase distress through their reactions. They can also be supporters to other bystanders. Bystanders can also play a role as witnesses and may be interviewed by law enforcement or be required to testify in court or in campus judicial procedures (Buzawa and Austin 1993; Shernock 2005). Bystanders can be "resisters" or "dissenters." We know from research that risk factors for SV and IPV include peer and cultural norms that support the use of coercion in relationships. Dissenters are those who actively speak out against these norms, challenging, for example, comments like the use of the term "rape" to describe a difficult exam in school. These bystanders exercise media literacy and use their voices to challenge media images of interpersonal violence as well as harassing comments (Ryan et al. 2006). Indeed, changing social norms requires in part these dissenting messages from multiple people who model a different descriptive norm—that not all people agree with rape myths or support violence and aggression—in a community, and who can work to change media coverage of stories on SV and IPV that influence how people think about these issues (Bowen et al. 2004; Franiuk et al. 2008). A related role is bystanders as spokesperson/trendsetter. In this role bystanders are change agents or change leaders. They actively pursue more education and awareness about SV and IPV, not just being reactive and responding to problematic situations but demonstrating support for violence prevention—displaying images such as slogans supporting violence prevention, posting positive stories about bystander action on social networking sites, talking to friends, family members, one's children about what healthy relationships are, encouraging community leaders to make statements related to violence prevention, volunteering for violence prevention or at agencies that support victims. These are the group of "innovators and early adopters" discussed by Rogers (2002) as the 15 % of people who embrace new ideas ahead of others and become role models for new community norms not just reacting against old ones. It is likely that the correlates of these different roles and the pros and cons of being in these roles will differ.

Lacking cognitive frameworks for how to help that work across these roles and actions may leave even motivated defenders immobilized. Understanding this conceptual mismatch between the way we usually think about helping and the resources we draw upon to do so and the helping scripts we need for sexual and relationship violence may provide new ideas for prevention. As will be discussed further below and in next chapters of this book, one solution to the mismatch of helping scripts is to ensure that prevention strategies include time to articulate and practice new helping scripts that can be flexibly used across bystander roles.

4.3.2 Emphasizing Relational Components of Bystander Action

Just as victims often know their perpetrators, given the context of SV and IPV, bystanders often know victims, perpetrators or both. In several studies of SV the position of the bystander in relation to the victim and perpetrator makes a difference for potential bystanders themselves in terms of attitudes and intention to help (Bennett et al. 2014). Bystanders, according to this work, are considering their position in relation to who needs help or who is creating the risky situation (Nicksa 2014). This raises key questions for our model of bystander action including: What do we need to add to a model that mostly describes helping strangers rather than helping friends? How do we better understand the impact of consequences of bystander actions given their connections to those involved and how those consequences (positive and negative) impact future attitudes and behaviors?

4.3.2.1 Creating New Scripts and Harnessing Potential Over Time: Moving Beyond Linear Views of Bystander Action

Helping in situations of SV and IPV may not be a one point in time event. We know that friends are the most likely individuals to receive a disclosure of SV (Banyard et al. 2010). Friends or family members may witness abuse consisting of many different incidents and behaviors and patterns of control over time in a relationship. Friends and family interviewed in one study described a process of becoming aware of the abuse in the relationship, trying different strategies to engage and help the victim, and even periods of disengagement from helping (Latta and Goodman 2011). Even sexual violence, which can be a single incident, may involve multiple occasions in which victims need help or support as they choose to disclose or not, seek formal services, or file a complaint with authorities. For example, a college student described the challenges of helping a friend in an abusive relationship, "Um well I've heard about it for a couple months now so like it's kind of hard to say the same things over and over and she doesn't seem to get the message but I still feel like I have to try to help her." There are multiple and yet linked opportunities for action by bystanders (Latta and Goodman 2011). While Latané and Darley's research does not describe helping specifically as linear, more recent uses of their work does seem to conceptualize this more step-wise path. We need to develop a model of bystander behavior as a process that may loop and coil over time to better account for the often relational context of bystander action in SV and IPV. We need a model that more transparently and intentionally describes the relationship between bystanders and other actors in the situation, between different correlates of bystander action and that follows these over time. Such a view could help potential bystanders anticipate these connections. For example, as noted in Chap. 3, we know very little about what is helpful to bystanders regarding helping friends.

From a research perspective we need more longitudinal studies of bystander action. How do actions link together over time? How often do bystanders help friends once with a single incident and how often does their helping consist of a series of actions over hours or days or months? Does the concept of linearity really apply or do bystanders find themselves going over and over the same actions, rather than through steps set out in a straight line? Do they revisit particular steps but not others as they help friends at different points along the continuum of risk for sexual assault? Research to date is relatively silent on these questions.

4.3.2.2 Bystander Behavior Doesn't End with Taking Action: Starting to See Consequences

Very little is currently understood about the impact of helping, both intended (did the action help?) and unintended (did the bystander get hurt or experience retaliation of some kind?). The relational nature of action to address SV and IPV foregrounds the issue of consequences. While Ullman (2010) has extensively studied victims' perspectives of reactions they receive to disclosure, we do not know about victims' perceptions of the range of bystander actions, nor have we studied bystanders' own perceptions of what happened once they intervened. Did they make the situation better? Did they make it worse? Did the identified victim feel positive about receiving help? Did the identified perpetrator retaliate? What about others who might have observed what went on and who might support the bystander or retaliate against them? Research on bystander behavior has considered how bystanders weigh potential pros and cons to stepping in as well as investigating barriers to action and highlighting types of helping that are likely to carry negative effects (Banyard 2008; Bennett et al. 2014; Dovidio et al. 1991; Osswald et al. 2010). These barriers or costs, however, have been studied mainly as *perceptions* of consequences or *anticipated* consequences when we talk about consequences at all and even these have not been well catalogued. We know little about describing actual consequences or how a bystander's status or position may influence those. For example, what are the actual negative and positive results of bystander action? As one student in my own study of bystander behavior remarked, "'What are people going to think about me?' Um, you know, 'What if the people involved know my friends so they're going to talk about me?' So, definitely self-image, what other people think about you, um, I think just fear is a big thing and just not wanting to get involved. Not wanting to get into a mess." Another stated, "I kinda have just a really strong trust with the majority of my friends and I also don't want them to be harmed so I would put myself out there for a friend but on a stranger, I would really, I would be a little hesitant only in the sense that I would wanna scan the situation to make sure that I would not be put in harm."

While bystanders in many situations may have questions about consequences, there are also likely unique consequences for SV and IPV that have not been well explored. Discussions of moral courage note that what distinguishes this form of helping are the potential negative consequences for bystanders but what those consequences look like are not specified (Osswald et al. 2010). One of the few studies of bystanders and multiple forms of victimization found that bystanders can be harmed by stepping in. Sexual assaults seemed to incur higher rates of bystander harm compared to other forms of victimization at least as reported by victims (Hamby et al. 2015). What is more, bystanders to SV and IPV may be more likely to know the victims and perpetrators involved in the situation since SV and IPV is most often perpetrated by someone the victim knows and in social and neighborhood contexts where bystanders are known as well. These relationships raise the stakes as bystanders may experience including harm to friendships, working relationships, or team unity.

We still know little about what bystander actions are the best to include in someone's skill set. Better understanding consequences of bystander actions will permit a more nuanced approach to training bystanders as potential prevention allies and helping bystanders stay safe from physical harm and other consequences (including more emotional consequences to relationships, socials standing, or sanctions by the community for a bystander's own behavior such as underage drinking). For example, one college student noted; "They were fighting it was late at night and he-he got very physical with her and at that point just kind of like "hey", you know, "are you alright?" And um I was walking towards them anyways to go past and um yeah I stepped in between them and um then they started turning on me...so I just kinda I-I walked away and called the campus cops. The girl initially turned around and said uh you know don't help me...That kind of made me kind of question whether or not I should of done it."

Future research is needed to answer the following questions: What negative and positive thoughts do bystanders have not only before taking action but while taking action? How did the people directly involved (the victim and perpetrator) react? Was the victim relieved? Was the perpetrator angry? What were the reactions of other bystanders in the situation? Were they supportive? Dismissive? Did they have a negative reaction to the bystander trying to help? How did the situation turn out? Was harm avoided for the victim? Did anyone get in trouble? Was a relationship damaged? Were supportive or derogatory social media posts made? Did the bystander end up being interviewed or called as a witness to a crime? Most importantly, how does experiencing any of these consequence then feed back into future decisions to take bystander action or not?

4.3.3 Embracing a Larger Ecological Model: Revisiting Community and Cultural Factors that Influence Bystander Actions

A revised model explaining bystander action also needs to more intentionally consider context. We know that a variety of community factors are a part of why violence happens and community interventions need to be part of the prevention equation (Casey and Lindhorst 2009; Pinchevsky & Wright, 2012). We also know that pro-social behavior or general helping is influenced by broader cultural and societal factors that are not captured in the microcosm of the immediate helping situation. For example, levels of helping differ by country and culture, by rural versus urban areas (see Banyard 2011 for a review: Pozzoli et al. 2012). More specific to bystander action and relationship abuse, actions are higher in communities with greater resources and greater collective efficacy (Edwards et al., 2014). At the more micro-level, teacher and school attitudes and parent and peer norms affect bystander behavior for bullying, and students are more likely to report a risk of violence on campus if they have greater trust in campus authorities (Hektner and Swenson 2012; Pozzoli and Gini 2012; Sulkowski 2011). For example, tests of Latané and Darley's situational model among primary and middle school students for defending against bullying showed the need for an expanded model to explain patterns in the data (Pozzoli and Gini 2013). In particular, inclusion of measures of peer and parent norms were important such that perceived pressure from parents and peers to help support victims predicted both attitudes and actions to defend the victims (see also Rigby and Johnson 2006).

How can we expand our understanding of the context of bystander intervention to better include different communities and ecological niches? In chapters two and three we saw how bystander research has looked mainly at the intra-individual and relational levels of the social-ecological model or the theory of triadic influence. We have done little to really investigate other aspects of context that might matter. Exploring these questions and their potential answers provides the foundation for an expanded model of bystander action. There are three components of a closer consideration of context for bystander action. The first is a consideration of the relationship of the individual bystander to his or her community and how the intersection of her/his identities in that community create different potential consequences or action choices (for example, is the bystander underage for drinking alcohol versus of legal age, is the bystander from an underrepresented group in that community?). The second is developmental context. The third is ecological niche or how cultural and community norms that may vary by ecological niche open possibilities or present restrictions for different bystander actions and how we help potential bystanders consider those.

4.3.3.1 Considering the Position of the Bystander: Social Position and Power not Just the Presence or Absence of Others

Knowing what to do or say and choosing to do so may depend on who the bystander is. As can be seen from the review of the bystander literature in the previous chapter, to date models of bystander action generally ignore the position/location or status of the bystander (one exception is Osswald et al. (2010) who discuss the social position of the bystander or type of government under which they act as aspects of moral courage but this discussion is not detailed and describes a more macro-sociological level than what I explore here). Whether the bystander is in the presence or absence of other bystanders is more often the focus of what is studied as is what is going on inside the head of the bystander. Some studies have considered the position of the victim (member of one's in-group or out-group, member of a racial minority) (Laner et al. 2001; Levine and Thompson 2004). Little considered is the position or status and power of the bystander themselves. In part this may come from the fact that early studies of bystander action were conducted around helping strangers, individuals who would be unlikely to know the status of the helper. Even in this literature clues exist about the relevance of social position. For example, researchers found greater defending by secondary school students with higher social status among their peers (Caravita et al. 2012). It may be easier to step in if one occupies a more high status or high power position, such as being older students on a college campus. In my own study, students described how a combination of experience, knowledge, but also power (e.g., being of legal age for drinking) contributed to this increased comfort. For example, "I definitely would be more willing [to help] than I used to be. I haven't been in many situations where that would come into play but I would be more than willing than I would freshman year… Being older comes with maturity completely." Another student remarked, "If I have any difference in opportunity to help, it's not because I'm older. It's because I've joined more clubs—I'm an officer in several clubs. I'm in more of a position of power so I can help."

To date, power, position, and status have been missing in a consideration of the context of bystander action in general and almost never explored in relation to sexual and relationship violence. There are many different ways that people can have power or be lacking in power. Bystanders have their own position in their communities—they have access to power or are lacking power in different circumstances given their membership in different social identity groups, their visibility as community leaders or not, how long they have been in the community. For example, in one research study about whether bystanders were likely to report child neglect, more highly educated community members and those in roles where they might come in contact with child maltreatment (teachers, medical professionals) were more likely to take action to address suspected child neglect (Fledderjohann and Johnson 2012). The impact of differences in position needs to be researched more carefully and a consideration of a bystander's position of power or lack of power should be thought through in prevention training.

For example, we can hypothesize that lack of access to power including being part of an underrepresented group in a community, presents particular barriers to helping because it may make a bystander vulnerable to more negative consequences. A bystander who is a member of an underrepresented group may step in but then be erroneously labeled as part of the problem or one of the perpetrators. A bystander's position may make her or him more or less likely to be supported and joined by others in taking action. Thus, a bystander's position in his or her community likely impacts the range of action options that seem possible or safe. For example, what are the implications for students from underrepresented cultural groups who choose to step in on a campus that is predominantly Caucasian? How are sexual minority students supported or seen as bystanders? Are individuals from marginalized groups or underrepresented groups at risk for more negative consequences or retaliation within the community when they step out as bystanders? Are they less likely to be supported by others? Are they more likely to be mistaken for being perpetrators rather than bystanders? What is more, a bystander's position in the community likely influences their sense of trust in other community members and in formal community helpers. To the extent that a bystander feels isolated or marginalized, they may be less likely to call police or campus authorities to help, or may feel less able to call on other community members to join with them in taking action. One study of college students found students with lower trust in campus authorities were less likely to say they would report suspicions of violence on campus (Sulkowski 2011).

4.3.3.2 Including a More Thorough Consideration of Time as Part of Bystander Action Processes

We also need a more developmental view. We may ask, what set of variables or resources, perhaps collected earlier in the lifespan, are needed to form the foundation for bystander action that may be taken later? How do we take a view of bystander action as well as a view of prevention that extends across the lifespan? Do bystander behaviors and the variables that impact them look different across the lifespan? Research suggests that helping skills develop over time, are influenced by developmental contexts like parenting (Carlo et al. 1999) and that certain aspects of bystander prevention may be more or less appropriately developmentally timed. Related to bullying, bystander intervention training seems to be more effective for high school students rather than younger students (Polanin et al. 2012). Is this finding due to age or developmental effects or is it that older high school students have higher social status and are more embedded in their communities? One college student described it this way, "I do feel a little more… Due to my experiences, I do feel like I'm a little more easily swayed to help a situation… I do feel more comfortable intervening after four years of being here [on campus]." How do we explain these developmental trajectories and how does that help us potentially link strategies to develop active bystanders over time?

We can start with a broad developmental question—how do we learn how to help? It seems to come in part from family contexts, we learn from our parents and caregivers; positive supportive parenting has been linked to prosocial tendencies (Carlo et al. 1999), is also linked to empathy and perspective taking (Espelage et al. 2012) and to moral development (Thornberg and Jungert 2013). Indeed, researchers of child development discuss the importance of early nurturing contexts for prosocial behavior (Biglan et al. 2012) while others talk about educational contexts that promote social and emotional learning (SEL) (Dulak et al. 2011). Studies show that SEL skills can be taught and are especially effective when taught by classroom teachers—perhaps because there is more diffusion of the innovation when actual school personnel are trained to do it (the personnel are then trained and may alter other aspects of classroom and their work, not just the curriculum presented to the students on SEL) (Durlak et al. 2011). This work suggests that we start developing active bystanders early rather than waiting until late adolescence or early adulthood.

Research also considers how bystander action may look different at different points in time, though the variety of measures used and variables studied makes comparisons challenging. We can also ask how correlates of helping may change over time. Studies of defenders in bullying showed the importance of moral responsibility, which might be similar or linked to to the sense of responsibility found by those who study college students (Banyard and Moynihan 2011; Pozzoli and Gini 2013). Children in middle school samples also showed effects of peers on bystander action, similar to the peer influences found among college students (Fabiano et al. 2003; Brown et al. in press; Pozzoli and Gini 2013). These results suggest patterns of developmental similarity in the correlates of helping. However, studies also show that models of defending behavior among bystanders to bullying did not fit younger children and adolescent samples equally well suggesting developmental differences (Pozzoli and Gini 2013). There is still much we need to understand about how our models of bystander action may look similar or may need to be different across the lifespan.

4.3.3.3 Ecological Niche: Community Norms for How it is Appropriate to Help

Finally, chapter three summarizes a few studies that support cross-cultural differences in quantity of helping. What is less understood is how communities and cultures vary in how helping happens or in what types of helping actions are seen as most appropriate. Prevention programs involve limited time to train participants. Thus, better tailoring the bystander action strategies that are practiced and demonstrated in prevention programs to match the range of options that are culturally salient to particular communities might increase prevention effectiveness. One ecological niche variable that has been more studied is gender and it can serve as an interesting example. We know from research that women and men often differ in what sort of situations they feel most comfortable helping in. In my own prevention work I have found, for example, that women discuss using distraction or distancing to address a risky situation while young men describe more direct intervention. In spite of actions they have taken in the past, young women ask for more opportunities to practice skills in prevention sessions to build confidence as active bystanders. On the other hand, young men need more encouragement to develop and use skills for diffusing, distancing, or delegating rather than just directly jumping into a situation that could be unsafe.

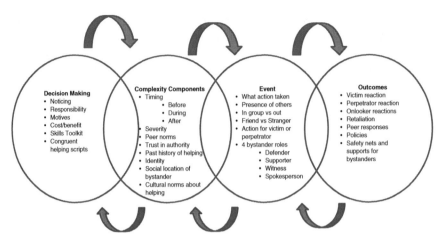

Fig. 1 Bystander action coils

4.4 Re-envisioning a Model of Bystander Behavior: From Helping Factors to Bystander Action Coils

Prevention efforts will be improved to the extent that we can better hone bystander action skills by being able to map out bystander actions that are most likely to be helpful and to minimize danger and costs to all in situations across different ecological niches. The process of helping can be expanded by envisioning notions of feedback loops, what I describe as bystander action coils, instead of a linear, single incident series of steps or stages (Chaudoir & Fisher 2010). The analogy of coils can better describe bystanders who help individuals with whom they have relationships over time and across situations. I draw this notion of process, and organization of some of its components from work by researchers confronting similar limitations in understanding how people choose to disclose or conceal a stigmatized identity (which includes the identity as a victim of SV or IPV) (Chaudoir & Fisher 2010). While Chaudoir and Fisher's model is specific to disclosure, not bystander action, it provides an interesting scaffolding for an expanded bystander model. I draw also from the Haddon Matrix model for analyzing injury prevention in public health (Barnett et al. 2005; Runyan 1998, 2003). The Haddon Matrix visually outlines a number of key dimensions of prevention including a consideration of factors across the ecological model (intra-individual variables, aspects of the person or vehicle of the problem, aspects of the immediate physical situation, and broader norms that make up the social context) and across time before, during, and after the injury event. Figure 4.1 presents a picture of what a revised model of bystander action could look like. The model blends work from across research on helping and bystander action in general with SV and IPV specific research. It more intentionally describes a process model of bystander action. It borrows the organizing framework from Chaudoir and Fisher (2010) and from the Haddon Matrix

(Runyan 2003) but adapts it for cataloguing in greater detail the additional components of helping that make bystander action for SV and IPV so complex.

The revised bystander action coil model includes specifications of the decision making process; contextual factors that impact decision processes as well as how the event may be related to outcomes; characteristics of the event itself; and outcomes of bystander action. Each of these represent a loop in the coil of bystander action and these loops potentially repeat over time developmentally as new skills and experiences are added to one's resources, attitudes, and behavior toolkit. The idea of multi-component loops allows for more clear specification of additional factors like the bystander's social position and context that while likely relevant to all bystander actions, are made particularly salient when considering SV and IPV. The first loop of the coil (action coil 1) represents an individual's internal decision making process. It is reviewed in detail in Chapter three as it includes the key components from previous bystander research using the situational model and in this way is not new (Latané and Darley 1970). This includes both the who of bystanders as well as motivations or why people help (to promote relationships or to act in a moral way that a person sees is "right," to improve one's self esteem or contribute to one's sense of self as a helpful person) or avoid action (desire to avoid risk to safety, to relationships). This component also includes an analysis of costs and benefits also described in other models (Dovidio et al. 1991) including consideration of barriers that are specific to SV and IPV situations (Bennett et al. 2014; Burn, 2009).

A variety of contextual variables or processes, the second action coil, can also be described and are in need of more research. This coil includes many of the factors described above as key components of an expanded model of bystander action that comes from research on SV and IPV. For example, perceived peer norms, whether related to the acceptance of coercion in relationships or norms about the appropriateness of helping, impact bystander action (Brown et al. in press; Brown and Messman-Moore 2010; Fabiano et al. 2003). Cultural norms and contexts are an extension of this and also impact individual decisions about whether and how to help (Pozzoli et al. 2012) and need to be a more explicit part of models of bystander behavior. They are included in this contextual processes coil. Expanding beyond friend norms, perceived relationships with community leaders, particularly trust in authorities may also make it more likely that bystanders will enlist the help of formal helpers such as school administrators (Sulkowski 2011), though to date we know little about what promotes this trust. The perceived severity of the situation also seems to impact attitudes and behavior (Bennett et al. 2014; Fisher et al. 2006) as are a bystanders' own past experiences with helping. This action coil should also include a consideration of the social position of the bystander. The position of the bystander connects to other coils in that it likely impacts all aspects of the decision process, mediating processes, and how the event itself unfolds.

The next component in the model (action coil 3: the event) is the coil that makes up the event itself. This encompasses the how of bystander action—what individuals choose to do and how they choose to act. Finally, this component also includes a consideration of the when and where or the context of the situation—the position of the bystander (how much power do they have in the situation?

In the broader community?), the number of bystanders present and the extent to which these bystanders know one another (Levine and Thompson 2004). It includes relationships among the parties in the situation, such that a bystander may feel safer to intervene if they know both parties but more likely to help if they only know the victim (Bennett et al. 2014). This coil also takes into account that bystanders play different roles depending on the type of SV and IPV they encounter (McMahon and Banyard 2012).

Finally, the fourth coil is about the outcomes of bystander action. This coil includes both current outcomes in the proximal situation but also past experiences of bystander action that likely impact choices and actions in the present. We need to know much more about the consequences of bystander action for victims (are they helped? Harmed?); for perpetrators (do they stop their behaviors? Is their behavior sanctioned in some way? If so, by whom or what?); and for bystanders (are they retaliated against for their actions?). Hamby et al. (2015) found that having a helpful bystander present was associated with more positive mental health outcomes for victims but that these positive effects were also more likely reported by victims if bystanders were not perceived as having been harmed. Indeed victim outcomes were less associated with the presence or absence of a bystander and more about whether the victim perceived that the bystander was harmed by being in the situation. Hart and Miethe (2008) conducted interesting analyses of helping ratios. They examined in what contexts across different types of crime bystanders are likely to be most helpful. For example, high helping ratios were for robberies and sex offenses that took place in daylight and involved strangers. Having a model that specifies consequences can promote further research on questions like: How do bystanders' past experience of helping affect present and future action? Are bystanders who experience negative reactions from victims, perpetrators or onlookers less likely to help in the future? Are they likely to keep helping but try a different type of action? What actions produce high positive outcomes for SV and how do these differ for IPV?

More information about all of these coils, and placing what we know about bystander correlates together in this process model will enable us to better train and advise potential bystanders about costs and benefits of helping, how best to evaluate their own safety, and generate actions that may work from their particular location.

4.5 Key Points Summary

- Research on bystander action often implicitly describes it as a linear process.
- Missing from current research is in-depth consideration of how helping unfolds and changes over time, including how consequences impact future helping.
- Examining instances of SV and IPV that bystanders confront makes clear that the relational context of helping is important.

4.5 Key Points Summary 71

- While the social-ecological model is a foundation for violence prevention work, the broader levels of bystanders' ecology have been less considered.
- The current chapter creates a new scaffold for bystander action research, "Bystander Action Coils," that is likely applicable to all forms of bystander helping but better nests all of the factors that we know are particularly important for SV and IPV responses.

4.6 Practice Implications

A number of practice implications and questions follow from this expanded model of bystander action. It calls for practices that consider the position of the bystander, developmental trajectories, and broader community contexts. Many of these will be more fully addressed in Chapters five and six. First, the new model suggests that we should talk to prevention participants about action as a process that may look different in the case of sexual and relationship violence from what they usually think of and do for helping. We must help participants anticipate these differences and identify new skills and scripts they may need to have. Helping is a process that may require periods of engagement and disengagement as friends experiencing SV or IPV may need different things at different times.

We need to understand much more about the outcomes of bystander actions, including negative repercussions and the variables that might mediate these outcomes. Are certain groups of people in a community more or less likely to be supported for taking bystander action? These topics can be part of discussions when training bystanders. Bystanders may need space to come back and have conversations about negative consequencees they experienced or actions they tried that were more or less successful. Following from this, we need to ask what more we should be doing to provide ongoing support and safety nets for bystanders. We know that helping in the context of sexual violence and relationship abuse is complicated, what policies and community resources can support these actions? Bystanders need the chance to build skills over time but also to loop back, check back in and discuss and receive support and further training once action has been tried and consequences experienced. This requires more than one-time training.

More linear bystander models that focus on getting potential bystanders from awareness to action (even if some looping back in thought processes happens in the middle) translate into prevention programs that are more closed ended, one point in time trainings. What the action coils model suggests instead is that we need to move from encouraging bystander action to cultivating bystander tenacity. Instances of relationship abuse or stalking intervention may take time. Many different actions may need to be tried over time and bystanders will not meet with success each time. We do not want bystanders to become discouraged especially since successes may not be clearly visible. We want bystanders to think about helping as a process over time, to think about meeting victims or potential victims where they are in one moment while being prepared to help again. Prevention resources need spaces to connect back with bystanders over time after initial education efforts. Ongoing training fits better with an action coils model.

We seem to assume that bystander intervention is helpful. But this may not always be the case (Hamby et al. 2015; Planty, 2002). Bystanders may take action that is not helpful to victims or actions that bring retaliation or negative consequences onto themselves or other bystanders. An expanded bystander model sets the stage for research on consequences of bystander actions so that our prevention efforts can more carefully advise potential bystanders about how they may best be helpful, how they can best minimize risks to themselves and others rather than taking the approach of just increasing action at all costs. We need to see which programs already include discussions of bystander safety in their programs (i.e. Eckstein et al. 2014) and whether what they are doing is enough or if the focus on safety ought to be a more expanded part of programming. This is especially important as more and more online bystander programs are created where direct interaction with participants is reduced and as campuses are mandated to include some form of bystander training in response to amendments to the federal Violence Against Women Act legislation.

We need to recognize that bystander action does not take place in a vacuum. It is impacted by contexts including community norms and policies. We should be attending as much to making changes in those areas as we are to changing the skills of individual bystanders (Lippy & DeGue 2014). Bystander action, like any other pro-social behavior, also does not come about overnight. It must be built on a foundation of positive development that can be strengthened by interconnected prevention efforts across the lifespan (Banyard 2013; Hamby and Grych 2013). For example, Peer Solutions (Peer Solutions 2010) takes a comprehensive, youth development approach to prevention that builds to bystander action through a series of interconnected protective factor strengthening components not all of which are bystander focused. More detail on specific prevention implications are discussed in chapters five and six. The purpose of this chapter was to show how an expanded model of bystander action in relation to sexual violence and relationship abuse can improve the logic models we use to describe both why we think bystander prevention may work and what components of our prevention tools are needed for it to be effective.

References

Avery, D. R., Richeson, J. A., Hebl, M. R., & Ambady, N. (2009). It does not have to be uncomfortable: The role of behavioral scripts in black–white interracial interactions. *Journal of Applied Psychology, 94*, 1382–1393.

Banyard, V. L. (2008). Measurement and correlates of pro-social bystander behavior: The case of interpersonal violence. *Violence and Victims, 23*, 85–99.

Banyard, V. L. (2011). Who will help prevent sexual violence: Creating an ecological model of bystander intervention. *Psychology of Violence, 1*, 216–229.

Banyard, V. L. (2013). Go big or go home: Reaching for a more integrated view of violence prevention. (Peer reviewed commentary). *Psychology of Violence, 3*, 115–120.

References

Banyard, V. L., & Moynihan, M. M. (2011). Variation in bystander behavior related to sexual and intimate partner violence prevention: Correlates in a sample of college students. *Psychology of Violence, 1*, 287–301.

Banyard, V. L., Moynihan, M. M., Walsh, W. A., Cohn, E. S., & Ward, S. K. (2010). Friends of survivors: The community impact of unwanted sexual experiences. *Journal of Interpersonal Violence, 25*, 242–256.

Barnett, D. J., Balicer, R. D., Blodgett, D., Fews, A. L., Parker, C. L., & Links, J. M. (2005). The application of the Haddon matrix to public health readiness and response planning. *Environmental Health Perspectives, 113*, 561–566.

Bennett, S., Banyard, V. L., & Garnhart, L. (2014). To act or not to act, that is the question? Barriers and facilitators of bystander intervention. *Journal of Interpersonal Violence, 29*, 476–496.

Biglan, A., Flay, B. R., Embry, D. D., & Sandler, I. N. (2012). The critical role of nurturing environments for promoting human well-being. *American Psychologist, 67*, 257–271.

Bowen, L. K., Gwiasda, V., & Brown, M. M. (2004). Engaging community residents to prevent violence. *Journal of Interpersonal Violence, 19*, 356–367.

Brown, A., & Messman-Moore, T. L. (2010). Personal and perceived peer attitudes supporting sexual aggression as predictors of male college students' willingness to intervene against sexual aggression. *Journal of Interpersonal Violence, 25*, 503–518.

Brown, A., Banyard, V. L., & Moynihan, M. M. (in press). The impact of perceived peer norms and gender, age, and race on bystander intentions and behaviors related to sexual violence. *Psychology of Women Quarterly*.

Burn, S. M. (2009). A situational model of sexual assault prevention through bystander intervention. *Sex Roles, 60*, 779–792.

Buzawa, E. S., & Austin, T. (1993). Determining police response to domestic violence victims. *The American Behavioral Scientist, 36*, 610–623.

Caravita, S. C. S., Gini, G., & Pozzoli, T. (2012). Main and moderated effects of moral cognition and status on bullying and defending. *Aggressive Behavior, 38*, 456–468.

Carlo, G., Fabes, R. A., Laible, D., & Kupanoff, K. (1999). Early adolescence and prosocial/moral behavior II: The role of social and contextual influences. *Journal of Early Adolescence, 19*, 133–147.

Casey, E. A., & Lindhorst, T. P. (2009). Toward a multi-level, ecological approach to the primary prevention of sexual assault: Prevention in peer and community contexts. *Trauma, Violence, and Abuse, 10*, 91–114.

Chan, S. (2007). "Gray rape": A new form of date rape? The New York Times, 22 Oct 2007.

Chaudoir, S. R., & Fisher, J. D. (2010). The disclosure process model: Understanding disclosure decision making and postdisclosure outcomes among people living with a concealable stigmatized identity. *Psychological Bulletin, 136*, 236–256.

Dovidio, J. F., Piliavin, J. A., Gaertner, S. L., Schroeder, D. A., & Clark, R. D. (1991). The arousal: Cost-reward model and the process of intervention: A review of the evidence. *Prosocial behavior: Review of personality and social psychology, 12*, 86–118.

Durlak, J. A., Weissberg, R. P., Dymnicki, A. B., Taylor, R. D., & Schellinger, K. B. (2011). The impact of enhancing students' social and emotional learning: A meta-analysis of school-based universal interventions. *Child Development, 82*, 405–432.

Eckstein, R., Moynihan, M. M. Banyard, V. L. & Plante, E. G. (2014). *Bringing in the bystander: A prevention workshop for establishing a community of responsibility*. Facilitator's Guide. Durham, NH: University of New Hampshire.

Edwards, K. & Banyard, V. (2014). *All helping is not equal: Rural young adults speak about sense of community and bystanders to relationship abuse*. Manuscript in preparation.

Edwards, K., Mattingly, M. J., Dixon. K. J., & Banyard, V. L. (2014). Community matters: Intimate partner violence among young adults. *American Journal of Community Psychology, 53*, 198–207.

Edwards, K., Mattingly, M. J., Dixon. K. J., & Banyard, V. L. (2014). Community matters: Intimate partner violence among young adults. *American Journal of Community Psychology, 53*, 198–207.

Espelage, D., Green, H., & Polanin, J. (2012). Willingness to intervene in bullying episodes among middle school students: Individual and peer-group influences. *The Journal of Early Adolescence, 32*, 776–801.

Fabiano, P. M., Perkins, H. W., Berkowitz, A., Linkenbach, J., & Stark, C. (2003). Engaging men as social justice allies in ending violence against women: Evidence for a social norms approach. *Journal of American College Health, 52*, 105–112.

Fischer, P., Greitemeyer, T., Pollozek, F., & Frey, D. (2006). The unresponsive bystander: Are bystanders more responsive in dangerous emergencies? *European Journal of Social Psychology, 36*, 267–278.

Fischer, P., Krueger, J. I., Greitemeyer, T., Vogrincic, C., Kastenmuller, A., & Frey, D. (2011). The bystander-effect: A meta-analytic review on bystander intervention in dangerous and non-dangerous emergencies. *Psychological Bulletin, 132*, 517–537.

Fledderjohann, J., & Johnson, D. R. (2012). What predicts the actions taken toward observed child neglect? The influence of community context and bystander characteristics. *Social Science Quarterly, 93*, 1030–1052.

Flood, M., & Pease, B. (2009). Factors influencing attitudes to violence against women. *Trauma, Violence, & Abuse, 10*, 125–142.

Frainuk, R., Seefelt, J. L., & Vandello, J. A. (2008). Prevalence of rape myths in headlines and their effects on attitudes toward rape. *Sex Roles, 58*, 790–801.

Goodman, L. A., & Epstein, D. (2011). The justice system response to domestic violence. In M. P. Koss, J. W. White, & A. E. Kazdin (Eds.), *Violence against women and children* (Vol. 2, pp. 215–235)., Navigating solutions Washington, DC, US: American Psychological Association.

GreenDot, Etc. (2015). An overview of the Green Dot strategy. http://www.calcasa.org/wp-content/uploads/2011/04/Curriculum-Summary.pdf. Accessed from 4 Mar 2015.

Hamby, S., & Grych, J. (2013). *The web of violence: Exploring connections among different forms of interpersonal violence and abuse*. The Netherlands: Springer.

Hamby, S., Weber, M., Grych, J. & Banyard, V. (2015). What difference do bystanders make? The association of victim outcomes with bystander involvement in a community sample.

Hart, T. C., & Miethe, T. D. (2008). Exploring bystander presence and intervention in nonfatal violent victimization: When does helping really help? *Violence and Victims, 23*, 637–651.

Hektner, J. M., & Swenson, C. A. (2012). Links from teacher beliefs to peer victimization and bystander intervention: Tests of mediating processes. *Journal of Early Adolescence, 32*, 516–536.

Janson, G. R., & Hazler, R. J. (2004). Trauma reactions of bystanders and victims to repetitive abuse experiences. *Violence and Victims, 19*, 239–255.

Laner, M. R., Benin, M. H., & Ventrone, N. A. (2001). Bystander attitudes toward victims of violence: Who's worth helping? *Deviant Behavior, 22*, 23–42.

Latané, B., & Darley, J. M. (1970). *The unresponsive bystander: Why doesn't he help?*. New York, NY: Appleton-Century-Crofts.

Latta, R. E., & Goodman, L. A. (2011). Intervening in partner violence against women: A grounded theory exploration of informal network members' experiences. *The Counseling Psychologist, 39*, 973–1023.

Levine, M., & Thompson, K. (2004). Identity, place, and bystander intervention: Social categories and helping after natural disasters. *The Journal of Social Psychology, 144*, 229–245.

Lippy, C., & DeGue, S. (2015). Exploring alcohol policy approaches to prevent sexual violence perpetration. *Trauma, Violence, & Abus*. Published online first.

McGregor, J. (2005). *Is it rape? On acquaintance rape and taking women's consent seriously*. Burlington, VT: Ashgate Publishing Company.

McMahon, S., & Banyard, V. L. (2012). When can I help? A conceptual framework for the prevention of sexual violence through bystander intervention. *Trauma, Violence, and Abuse, 13*, 3–14.

McMahon, S., Banyard, V. & McMahon, S. (2015). Incoming college students' bystander behaviors to prevent sexual violence. *Journal of College Student Development, 56*, 488–493.

Nicksa, S. C. (2014). Bystander's willingness to report theft, physical assault, and sexual assault: The impact of gender, anonymity, and relationship with the offender. *Journal of Interpersonal Violence, 29*, 217–236.

Osswald, S., Greitemeyer, T., Fischer, P., & Frey, D. (2010). What is moral courage? Definition, explication, and classification of a complex construct. In C. L. Pury & S. J. Lopez (Eds.), *The psychology of courage: Modern research on an ancient virtue* (pp. 149–164). Washington, D.C.: American Psychological Association.

Peer Solutions. (2010). *Stand & serve primary prevention evidence based research.* Retrieved from http://www.peersolutions.org/stand-and-serve

Pinchevsky, G. M., & Wright, E. M. (2012). The impact of neighborhoods on intimate partner violence and victimization. *Trauma, Violence, & Abuse, 13*(2), 112–132.

Planty, M. (2002). *Third-party involvement in violent crime, 1993–1999.* Bureau of justice statistics special report. Washington, D.C. U.S. Department of Justice. NCJ189100.

Polanin, J. R., Espelage, D. L., & Pigott, T. D. (2012). A meta-analysis of school-based bullying prevention programs' effects on bystander intervention behavior. *School Psychology Review, 41,* 47–65.

Pozzoli, T., & Gini, G. (2010). Active defending and passive bystanding behavior in bullying: The role of personal characteristics and perceived peer pressure. *Journal of Abnormal Child Psychology, 38,* 815–827.

Pozzoli, T., & Gini, G. (2012). Why do bystanders of bullying help or not? A multidimensional model. *Journal of Early Adolescence, 33,* 315–340.

Pozzoli, T., & Gini, G. (2013). Friend similarity in attitudes toward bullying and sense of responsibility to intervene. *Social Influence, 8,* 161–176.

Pozzoli, T., Ang, R. P., & Gini, G. (2012). Bystanders' reactions to bullying: A cross-cultural analysis of personal correlates among Italian and Singaporean students. *Social Development, 21,* 686–703.

Rigby, K., & Johnson, B. (2006). Expressed readiness of Australian schoolchildren to act as bystanders in support of children who are being bullied. *Educational Psychology, 26,* 425–440.

Rogers, E. M. (2002). Diffusion of preventive innovations. *Addictive Behaviors, 27,* 989–993.

Runyan, C. W. (1998). Using the Haddon matrix: Introducing the third dimension. *Injury Prevention, 4,* 302–307.

Runyan, C. W. (2003). Introduction: Back to the future—revisiting Haddon's conceptualization of injury epidemiology and prevention. *Epidemiologic Reviews, 25,* 60–64.

Ryan, C., Anastario, M., & DaCunha, A. (2006). Changing coverage of domestic violence murders: A longitudinal experiment in participatory communication. *Journal of Interpersonal Violence, 21,* 209–228.

Shernock, S. (2005). Third party roles in intimate partner violence incidents and their effects on police response in a statewide rural jurisdiction. *Journal of Police and Criminal Psychology, 20,* 22–39.

Sulkowski, M. L. (2011). An investigation of students' willingness to report threats of violence in campus communities. *Psychology of Violence, 1,* 53–65.

Thornberg, R., & Jungert, T. (2013). Bystander behavior in bullying situations: Basic moral sensitivity, moral disengagement and defender self-efficacy. *Journal of Adolescence, 36,* 475–483.

Ullman, S. (2010). *Talking about sexual assault: Society's response to survivors.* Washington, DC: American Psychological Association.

White, C. H., & Malkowski, J. (2014). Communicative challenges of bystander intervention: Impact of goals and message design logic on strategies college students use to intervene in drinking situations. *Health Communication, 29,* 93–104.

Winerip, M. (2014). Stepping up to stop sexual assault. *New York Times Education Life,* 9 Feb 2014.

Chapter 5
Building a Better Bystander

> *A girl was really a mess and this guy wasn't pressuring her necessarily, but, um, you could kind of tell she just wasn't having it. She was not interested in his intentions at all and he was just being really overbearing and I just looked and jumped in the situation and made it super awkward. And the guy kind of got mad at me and then took off. It was a situation where I had fun with it anyway. It was actually one month after this program actually happened, when I was a freshman…when I was still kind of thinking about that all the time, you know?*
> —College student who participated in Bringing in the Bystander TM program during the first semester on campus

Abstract Bystander action related to sexual and relationship violence is not just about describing when someone will step into reduce the risk of an assault. Prevention strategies are about changing people's behavior to make it more likely that they will take safe action across a range of roles bystanders find themselves in. This chapter draws from research on attitude and behavior change in social psychology, health behavior, and research on prevention efficacy to outline a set of strategies and research questions across coils of bystander actions that may make bystander focused violence prevention more effective. These include strategies that focus first on attitudes, those that highlight behavior change more directly, and methods that change the broader community norms context in which bystanders act.

Keywords Prevention · Social norms · Behavior change · Persuasion

A key limitation of bystander research to date is that it mainly focuses on the who, when, and where of prosocial bystander action. Models of bystander behavior, as described in the previous chapters, seek mainly to describe hystander intervention— under what conditions it is likely to occur or not. Chapter 4 presented a revised model for tying these factors together through a framework of "action coils." This is a helpful foundation to leverage helpful bystander intervention or informal social control in communities. Indeed, current discussions of bystanders to sexual violence and relationship abuse have taken social psychological inquiry further by asking how we can we predict bystander action *and* change it? This chapter provides an overview and synthesis of what we know about change processes with applications to bystander action for sexual and relationship violence prevention. I use the model of action coils described in Chap. 4 as a way to organize these change strategies. It should be noted that each change strategy may well be effective for changing some aspect of more than one of the action coils. I have tried to discuss each change mechanism in the coil that seems most relevant to it. Each coil has different entry points for change, with some like the first focused on decision processes at the individual level and others addressing community or policy doorways.

5.1 Changing Action Coil 1: Influencing Individual Decision Making

As described in the previous chapter, action coil one derives mainly from previous theories of bystander action especially the situational model of Latané and Darley (1970). It consists of variables within the bystander including their appraisal of the situation and potential responses (e.g. awareness, sense of responsibility, and confidence to act which are also related to variables like victim blaming attitudes). Mechanisms for changing the elements of this coil come from research on health behavior change, experimental social psychology, and prejudice reduction. They share a focus on changing attitudes and behaviors, including those that are strongly believed in and are often outside of awareness. Change centers on individuals (e.g. attitudes about rape myths, perceptions of the value of helping, beliefs about community member's responsibility to one another, whether one acts to help someone, walks away or pulls out their phone to take a picture to share via social media). While we know that the link between attitudes and behaviors is not always strong, we do have evidence that it is an important connection to attend to. Recent research on bystander behaviors related to SV and IPV found, for example, that more gender equitable attitudes were related to greater intent to be a bystander and lower odds of perpetrating SV or IPV among high school boys (Das et al. 2012; McCauley et al. 2013). The researchers highlighted changing these sorts of ingrained gender attitudes as one important component of prevention work. Other research showed bystander confidence and intent to act were related to greater amounts of bystander behavior to address IPV and SV situations (Banyard 2008; Banyard and Moynihan 2011).

5.1.1 Changing Individual Attitudes

Persuasion is the term for techniques that focus on changing beliefs and attitudes first, assuming that behavior change will follow (Brown 2006; Zimbardo and Leippe 1991). We need to get new messages in front of potential bystanders and do so in engaging ways so that even more implicit and unacknowledged attitudes are brought into awareness to be examined. This can be challenging since humans often use filters that make us more attentive to messages that confirm and support what we already believe. Potential bystanders may be more or less open to messages encouraging action based on their prior attitudes and experiences with helping. Bystanders are likely to automatically pay attention to media stories that confirm beliefs they already have, that reinforce victim blaming for example or that leave bystanders out of the story or that highlight bystanders who do nothing. This suggests that presenting different information about bystander action—like showcasing an example of positive and helpful bystander intervention need to be presented often over time in order to better attract people's attention. Once an attention grabbing dose has been achieved, prevention messages may need to change frequently in order to continue to provide new information. Social marketing campaigns like "My Strength" (Men Can Stop Rape) or "Know Your Power" (Potter 2012) include a number of different images displayed in a community over time and often updated (Potter and Stapleton 2011).

Furthermore, we tend to see messages as being fairer and less biased based on the closer the messages are to what we already believe (see Brown 2006 for a review of social judgment theory). If a new message is too new and different from our foundation of attitudes, we are likely to reject it out of hand (Sherif et al. 1973). What is more likely to change attitudes is a series of messages that push people just a bit further each time, moving them toward more substantial changes via baby steps that do not seem too uncomfortable or new. This finding fits well with points made in Chap. 4 about the need for a developmental perspective. If we work incrementally toward changes in bystander actions, we will be more successful in promoting growth in prevention related attitudes in college. For example, if a solid foundation for these attitudes is formed earlier. As another example, a recently released film "Escalation" tells the story of relationship abuse and one young woman's murder by her partner while friends looked the other way or were insensitive to warning signs (One Love Foundation 2015). What is interesting is that the film starts with a dating relationship that seems to fit our usual ways of thinking about couples in college. Slowly the landscape changes as the relationship becomes more controlling and dangerous and potential bystanders realize their series of missed opportunities. The film begins with a story that fits with attitude systems but then presents new information, and in a dramatic fashion that asks for re-examination of how we think about what control by an intimate partner looks like and how bystanders can help. To date, however, prevention evaluation has mainly been on educational workshops with much less attention to the impact of films and social marketing campaigns as delivery methods for new messages (see Potter 2012 for an exception).

Another component of effective persuasion is the problem of distraction (Brown 2006). At any given moment several different messages or stimuli may be competing for our attention and make it difficult to process messages thoroughly. Instead of being influenced by the quality of the argument or information, we are affected by simply how many times the message is presented or by how attractive visual images displayed with the message are. This finding too has implications for prevention education. Bystander education is increasingly going online (For example, PETSA (2014) at the University of Montana, RealConsent (2014) at Emory University (Salazar et al. 2014), Take Care (Kleinsasser et al. 2015), Every Choice (2014) by GreenDot, Agent of Change (Schewe 2013), the National Sexual Violence Resource Center has an online bystander course, and Havens by Everfi (2014) describes including a bystander component). This has potential from a persuasion perspective in that messages can be put in front of individuals frequently (every year when they enroll in classes or sign up for campus housing, for example), can be attention grabbing through the use of videos and online skits, and can visually bring to awareness attitudes and beliefs. Indeed, some evaluations are promising about this approach (Kleinsasser et al. 2015; Salazar et al. 2014). Circle of Six is an app that allows an individual to instantly contact friends they have programmed in who can be called upon to pick them up from a risky situation, call them to check in, etc. (www.Circleof6app.com). As a phone app it is a stimulus that is constantly on display reminding friends about the power of bystander intervention. More evaluation research is needed about the effectiveness of these strategies.

On the other hand, online delivery of prevention gives participants messages in contexts over which prevention educators have little control—on their smartphones at a sporting event, in college residence halls surrounded by friends, or in the quiet of a library study room. Some settings present more distractions and barriers to central and deep processing of messages. Thus the question arises: How do we design accessible prevention tools to reach diverse audiences while also insuring that individuals pay careful attention to the messages we send? We need to make sure that the delivery mechanism doesn't dilute the power of prevention information. Research is needed and should include questions that ask participants where they took the online training and if they were alone or with others.

We also need to ensure that the individual is able to understand the message. We know from the science of teaching and learning that individuals learn new material best to the extent that it is connected to something they already know, is connected to personal experience (the self-reference effect), is presented in an organized way, and where learners have opportunities to use and practice the information rather than passively receive it (Zinkiewicz et al. 2003). Bystander messages in social marketing campaigns are more effective if people see the images as similar to them (Potter and Stapleton 2012). Bystander intervention is a framework that has been applied to many different community problems including drunk driving, suicidality, and violence prevention though not necessarily in the same location (Cimini et al. 2014; Guerette et al. 2013; Polanin et al. 2012). It is interesting to consider what might happen if bystander training and the use of this framework was employed to address a number of issues within a community. Then messages about taking action to help in situations of SV or IPV would not seem so new or different from existing information and skills that individuals have. In part this is what has made bystander intervention successful, that it builds on what people already know about helping. But as discussed in Chap. 4, bystander action for SV and IPV

5.1 Changing Action Coil 1: Influencing Individual Decision Making

is often quite different from general helping. Yet it has common threads in its complexity to helping a friend who has had too much to drink and wants to drive or helping someone in psychological distress. Working across issues using this common framework may enhance the effectiveness of our work (Banyard 2014).

We have much to learn about methods of message delivery. What do potential bystanders understand if information presented as part of a social marketing campaign, an online training, or an in-person discussion. What combination of delivery format is optimal (Banyard 2014)? Borges et al. (2008) found that university students showed a greater understanding of a campus consent policy when they were read the policy *and* given a chance to discuss it. Yet this is one of the few single studies to directly compare different teaching methods in the context of SV and IPV prevention. Indeed, the goal of prevention is to encourage deeper processing and understanding of messages rather than superficial acceptance or rejection (Heppner et al. 2001). Yet to date, most prevention work related to SV and IPV uses limited teaching methods with less emphasis on active skill building components (DeGue et al. 2014).

From a prevention standpoint research also supports the need for multiple messages over time (Nation et al. 2003) and messages that build on one another. In Chap. 4, I discussed a dynamic model of "action coils." In this model bystander action is a process over time, with earlier experiences connecting to later experiences. Individuals need repetition of information to learn it (not all at once but over time, Carpenter et al. 2012) and to strengthen the availability of the changed attitude so that it can quickly be accessed in a situation and thus have more influence over behavior (Brown 2006; Zimbardo and Leippe 1991; Boher and Dickel 2011). One study showed benefits of combining bystander training workshops with a social marketing campaign (Banyard et al. unpublished manuscript). Individuals may need different pieces of information at one point, and then new messages that take them further later on. To date, however, both our prevention strategies and our evaluation of their effectiveness have fallen short of examining such comprehensive ways of thinking. For example, when evaluating a prevention program it would be important to ask what previous experiences participants had with prevention both generally and specific to SV or IPV. We then need to analyze the impact of those previous learning experiences on what they got out of a current program. Such questions are rarely asked or analyzed.

Attitude change also involves creating positive associations with the new message (see Haines 1996; Glider et al. 2001 for research on the efficacy of positive norming messages to reduce substance use among young adults). We need strong and clear bystander messages that create positive associations with being a bystander and make sure the positive attitude is easy to translate into behavior. We should ask whether the prevention tools we use showcase positive aspects of being a bystander and benefits of attitude change rather than just presenting information about the problem. One program, Bringing in the Bystander™, has participants start by thinking of examples when they helped someone else with a positive result or when someone helped them. This creates a positive context for thinking about bystander action. A bystander focused social marketing campaign, Know Your Power™ (Potter

2012) displays examples of positive and safe bystander behaviors to address sexual and relationship violence. The idea is to make it easier for individuals who view the images to translate and incorporate the message into their own behavior. These suggestions have to date mainly focused on bystanders as defenders and supporters. As noted in earlier chapters, bystanders can also play other roles including dissenters and spokespeople. We need prevention messages that teach individuals how to have healthy conversations about consent, to understand what respectful egalitarian relationships look like and encourage their friends to have them since we know healthy relationships are more than the absence of violence and coercion and to actively display symbols and messages of support for nonviolence. Bystanders can in this way work to promote healthy communication skills, not just discourage rape myths. A recent prevention evaluation showed promising results from this integration of healthy sexuality with bystander intervention (Salazar et al. 2014).

Prevention strategies also need to help bystanders overcome barriers to stepping in. While we want bystanders to carefully consider their own safety when choosing when and how to act, we also want them to have courage in the face of worries about negative evaluations by others who see them step in. A line of research in social psychology suggests that narrative approaches—having people write or think about a time when they were powerful—reduces concerns about being negatively judged by others for one's actions (Schmid and Schmid Mast 2013). It is interesting to think about how exercises like this might be incorporated into bystander training and confidence building.

Ultimately, lasting attitude changes occurs when individuals take over the persuasion themselves, creating their own "self-generated arguments (Zimbardo and Leippe 1991, p. 181)." This active self-persuasion is encouraged by creating direct experience, opportunities to role play adopting different points of view and different behaviors. Studies show that when trying to help people overcome biased attitudes toward an issue or group, it is not effective to simply point out their biases and encourage them to think more critically. Instead, individuals can be asked to talk about how information might support a different position from their own, to take the position of someone with a different view (Paluck and Green 2009). Interactive theater makes use of this change mechanism (Ahrens et al. 2011; McMahon et al. 2011; Sex Signals) as audience members are encouraged to add their own ideas to the unfolding improvisational script performed by actions in scenes of escalating risk for sexual violence or what happens in its aftermath. Bringing in the Bystander™ is a bystander training curriculum that asks participants to generate their own bystander strategies and plan.

5.1.2 Changing Behavior First

Finally, we also know that creating a particular behavior that may be in conflict with attitudes can lead an individual to change their attitude through cognitive dissonance or hypocrisy salience (Paul and Gray 2011; Schumacher and Smith

Slep 2004). Going through the motions of helping creates a self-perception that one is a "helpful person" which then begins to instigate more helping behavior. This is why role playing (Zimbardo and Leippe 1991) is part of interactive theatre (Ahrens et al. 2011) and most bystander prevention programs. The essential element of this process is that there is a mismatch between different thoughts or views held within the same person or between a person's behavior and attitudes. This conflict creates unpleasant arousal. Paul and Grey (2011) talked about how individuals might be asked to prepare a public talk about the problem of sexual assault and the need for helpful bystanders while also being asked to think about a time when they used coercion or abused power in a relationship or failed to call out someone else who was.

Indeed the use of narrative and expressive writing as a component of prevention has been understudied and may be another way for potential bystanders to act out new ways of helping, by sharing writing with others, to publically commit to stepping in (Wilson 2011). I discuss this further below as a facet of action coil two and the problem of identity. Following the "commitment principle" (Zimbardo and Leippe 1991, p. 79), people who make some sort of more public declaration then feel responsible for following through. Bringing in the Bystander, a sexual violence prevention program for college campuses has all participants sign a bystander pledge—a public commitment to action within the prevention program. The White Ribbon Campaign is a more public form of committing to work to end violence. It is an example of the "do good, be good" approach which finds that getting people to do small actions can help them see themselves as the sort of person who does things like take action to prevent SV and IPV (Wilson 2011). As another example, playing prosocial video games which included rescuing or taking care of characters was associated with greater helping not just in the form of small kindnesses like picking up dropped pencils or volunteering to participate in a study, but stepping into help a young woman who was being verbally harassed and physically threatened by an ex-partner (Greitemeyer and Osswald 2010). Playing violent games was linked to reduced helping of someone harmed in a physical fight (Bushman and Anderson 2009). Perhaps embedding video games with helping components into bystander focused training would help to set in motion prosocial actions that will help individuals see themselves more as people who step into help in instances of SV and IPV. Indeed, a recent innovation in assessment of bystander behavior may also itself be a form of innovation—the use of virtual reality to put people in situations of being a bystander to SV and IPV and giving them a chance to take action (Jouriles et al. 2014). What is more, other researchers found that playing general video games cooperatively with another player promotes helping (Greitemeyer et al. 2012; Greitemeyer and Cox 2013; Velez et al. 2012). This suggests that online bystander training may want to include a cooperative game component where friends work together in scenarios. Perhaps this simulated cooperation will enhance supportive group contexts for taking bystander action. More research is needed on how encouraging small public behaviors or using simulated behaviors in games can set in motion action coils toward more bystander actions over time.

Other techniques may assist in overcoming barriers to action. One group of researchers was interested in trying to reduce the bystander effect (suppression of helping in the presence of others due to worries they will be judged negatively). Participants in a series of studies completed a writing task to disinhibit this behavioral control, a "disinhibition manipulation (van den Bos et al. 2009, p. 874)." Participants wrote about a time when they acted with "no inhibitions" and described what they did and how they felt. After this writing task people were more likely to help someone pick up a dropped item even in the presence of others. They also acted faster to help someone who was choking. While these are not the same helping contexts as IPV and SV, perhaps an exercise like this would be a good opening for bystander training workshops to reduce disinhibition as bystanders start learning and practicing challenging actions.

5.1.3 Using Interactions and Relationships to Change Attitudes

We can also look beyond strategies that focus on individuals to relational strategies that create change. Like groups and individuals marginalized based on their race, religion, or sexual orientation, victims of violence are often viewed negatively by others, blamed for their situation, and denied supports and resources (Chaudoir and Fisher 2010; Ullman 2010). Research continues to document that people see victims of SV and IPV as being to blame for their situations (because they were drinking, because of what they were wearing, because they did not leave the relationship) or they believe that victims falsely report instances of SV and IPV and thus do not believe what victims say when they come forward. Young men who hold more gender inequitable attitudes and see women as less than men are not only more likely to perpetrate SV and IPV but less likely to take action as bystanders (Das et al. 2012; McCauley et al. 2013). A number of strategies to address prejudice, including exercises to bring people in contact with the negatively perceived group and to see connections between themselves and these group members, have implications for decreasing bystanders' attitudes that are barriers to action and for building bystander motivation.

One intervention method, based on the contact hypothesis, brings together members of different groups who have equal status to work together on shared goals or to learn cooperatively as a way to reduce these prejudices (Paluck and Green 2009). Indeed, in the context of race-based bullying among adolescents, greater contact with underrepresented groups was linked to greater intent to take bystander action as a result of increased empathy, greater cultural openness and lesser favoritism towards one's own in-group (Abbott and Cameron 2014). This may not be easily translated to violence prevention research as victims understandably do not want to be identified as such. However, many advocacy and crisis centers do have survivors who are public about their experiences. These survivors often work with community members on common goals of violence prevention such as Take Back the Night marches. To date, however, we have little research on the effectiveness of these events. Prevention messages are also likely to be more effective to the extent that they include local stories to make it more real that both active bystanders and real victims are members of an individual's community. Bystanders and victims are the very people we have relationships with as friends, neighbors, family members, co-workers. For example, on one college campus in Texas they launched an awareness campaign titled "Remember Me" that featured the publically available names of local victims of relationship violence who were killed by their partners. The campaign created connections to victims who were part of a potential bystander's local community. Another project worked first with survivors of IPV to help them support and tell their stories to one another through photography but then connected survivors and their stories to the community through public exhibitions of their work (Frohmann 2005). An interesting line of work in prejudice reduction finds that even imagined contact with out-group members can be effective in improving attitudes (Crisp and Turner 2012). This suggests that simulation exercises using imagery could be a useful component of bystander work.

This work reminds us that interpersonal connections are a powerful and important part of the work of changing attitudes and behaviors, yet few prevention programs include relationship building and group work (DeGue et al. 2014). It is interesting that Safe Dates (Foshee et al. 2014) includes a component which involves participants working together to create a theatrical performance. Potential bystanders create something to change attitudes in their community. It would be interesting to assess the importance of the collaborative work as an ingredient in the program's effectiveness. Some school based programs make use of older students as models who can share their experiences with younger students (Katz et al. 2011) and Coaching Boys to Men uses relationships between coaches and their players to leverage attitude and behavior changes (Miller et al. 2012b).

Another component of mobilizing relationships centers on understanding how individuals see themselves in relation to others, noting that we need connections to others and to groups in order to help (Levine and Thompson 2004; Levine et al. 2005). The more we see ourselves as sharing an aspect of our identity with a person needing help, and the more that part of ourselves is front and center in our thinking at the moment, the more likely we are to take action. Researchers have been able to manipulate the prominence of different aspects of identity to increase responsibility to provide help. For example, activating one's sense of being a soccer fan in general rather than a fan of a specific team made it more likely you would help a fan of an opposing team if they were hurt (Levine and Thompson 2004; Levine et al. 2005). We can imagine how we might promote helping beyond looking out for friends by helping college students see themselves as members of the full campus community, rather than identifying particularly with a sub-community like a residence hall or a group of friends or a team. On the other hand, bystander programs may also work better when training is done within sub-communities of a town like a church, or a set of restaurant owners, or within professional groups like school principals in a district or region, to capitalize on in-group perceptions. Some school-based programs train bystanders within residence halls or by team (Gidycz et al. 2011). Many bystander trainings encourage participants to see victims of SV and IPV as family members or friends (Katz et al. 2011).

Communities need to find ways of building shared community identities so that bystanders see all citizens of their town or neighborhood, for example, as members of their in-group who deserve bystander action. These strategies may also help address problems with the social location of bystanders. The social position of a potential bystander (whether they are part of an underrepresented group for example) may present barriers or safety concerns. To the extent that more common community identities (we're all part of this organization or team) are activated, it may give less salience to these other aspects of the bystander and reduce negative consequences for bystanders. On the other hand, a component of bystander skill building could also involve helping potential bystanders identify aspects of their identity that hold more or less power in their community and teach ways to make the more powerful roles more salient when stepping in as a bystander. For example, a young woman might have more power as a bystander when wearing an athletic team jacket that advertises what might be perceived as a higher status role on campus. Bystanders should also be encouraged to take action with others rather than alone as group intervention will give support to bystanders and likely make less salient the power status of individual members. Building relationships between bystanders is yet another component of relationship-focused change strategies.

5.1.4 Addressing More Than One Attitude at a Time

Theories of health behavior change (including the Theory of Planned Behavior and Health Belief Model) have been the most often cited as foundations for violence prevention and a key lesson they offer is that we must be conscious of working to change several different attitudes at the same time (Abraham and Sheeran 2005; Ajzen 1991; Banyard 2014 for a review; Cox et al. 2010; Gidycz et al. 2001; Madden et al. 1992). We need to do a much better job of examining the different components of bystander action related attitudes together in research, to understand how they relate to one another but also to understand the extent to which some may be more powerful or important correlates of action. This would help us ensure that prevention efforts focus on the range of most central attitudes that should be changed to promote helping. We need comprehensive attitude change strategies that do more than just raise awareness, for example. That is only one component of the attitude system related to bystander action (Zimbardo and Leippe 1991). Prevention programs need to raise awareness and increase motivation to see SV and IPV as problems relevant to participants but also increase participants' sense of responsibility to act, and shift their perceptions that they have the knowledge and skills to act. Awareness must also be put to use in the development of skills and options for action (Nation et al. 2003; Wilson 2011). To date,

5.1.5 Accounting for Individual Differences in Attitude Change Approaches

Research is also clear that individuals vary in what change mechanisms will work best for them (see, for example, the transtheoretical model Grimley et al. 1994). We likely need different bystander prevention strategies to reach individuals at different levels of motivation or readiness to help with the problem of IPV and SV. For example, a person may start with no awareness that SV exists in her/his community and thus they have little motivation to do anything to address the problem. They will need more work on understanding how the problem impacts them and people they know, and building a sense of responsibility for doing something. They need exposure to community norms that support bystander action (Potter 2012). Someone in a later stage of readiness would benefit more from building specific skills for taking action (Banyard et al. 2010). College students who were at a higher level of readiness to change (they expressed more awareness of the problem of SV and IPV) before they received bystander prevention education, reported greater impact of the program on bystander actions (e.g., they self-reported performing more types of bystander actions to prevent sexual violence after the program) (Moynihan et al. 2015). To date, evaluation of SV and IPV prevention programs have rarely analyzed these types of moderators and they should be the focus of future research (Banyard 2014). Online prevention methods also hold promise here. They could provide gateway assessments of an individual's attitudes and readiness and then based on those results, direct participants to different bystander training modules that could be tailored to what they need to learn next.

Gender differences in bystander action suggest that men and women may need somewhat different bystander training (Leone et al. 2015). A consistent finding is that women have greater knowledge about SV and IPV and endorse fewer myths. They may need bystander programs that focus less on awareness and responsibility and more on safe intervention options. Men on the other hand may need both awareness building but also programs that focus on masculinity and expectations of masculine gender roles and how these can facilitate but also make bystander action more difficult.

Variability in prevention audiences also likely intersects with who provides prevention education. Attitude and behavior changes are more likely produced when knowledge and information are provided by credible and engaging sources of the message. Yet these credibility perceptions may differ by audience (Brown 2006). We know people are strongly motivated to be right and to have the right information to do the right thing in different situations. We look to credible others for information to help us with this ("informational influence", Brown 2006; Zimbardo and Leippe 1991). The Coaching Boys to Men program trains coaches as key information leaders for young athletes with promising results for SV and IPV prevention (Das et al. 2012; Miller et al. 2012b). There are somewhat mixed findings about who best to deliver SV and IPV prevention overall in meta-analyses with some studies finding support for peers and others for professionals. Yet, studies have not really directly compared the two groups using the same prevention program. Drawing conclusions about which message source is more effective is not yet possible. Such research should also look at variables within the audience that may interact with who the messenger is. Perhaps there are some audiences for whom peer facilitators work better and some who need to hear prevention from professionals. More information about these questions would be useful. To improve message quality we also need to have information about our audiences including their prior knowledge and experience. Rather than using prevention methods that have been copied and pasted from other communities, we must tailor our messages to each new community (Potter and Stapleton 2011), meet individual differences in knowledge and experience (Banyard et al. 2010) and more carefully explore the effectiveness of a range of trainers.

5.2 Changing Action Coil 2: Contextual Processes

Action coil two consists of contextual variables that surround and influence potential bystanders. Key variables include relationships with others, norms, and community connections. These forces may be best changed through policies, more comprehensive community strategies of change (Taylor et al. 2013; Wandersman and Florin 2003) or by bridging individual and community strategies in more micro/relational/interactional contexts such as peer norms (e.g. Paul and Gray 2011). This action coil helps us think beyond what is going on inside the head of the bystander, to factors that operate like grooves in the pavement to alert drivers they are going off the road rather than asking them not to drive when tired or water purification systems to change water quality rather than asking people to boil their water. For example, Taylor et al. (2013) documented the effectiveness of violence prevention that identified places in the school where violence and harassment were most likely to happen and repositioned staff there to oversee what was going on. Changing aspects of the context changed individual behaviors.

5.2.1 Change Community Leaders and Engage Early Adopters

The research related to action coil two suggests that a key leverage point for prevention is to start by changing people who surround individual bystanders. Several change theories highlight the need to focus on peer leaders who others look to for information, modeling, and norms (Kelly 2004; Rogers 2002; Staggs et al. 2007). Mentors in Violence Prevention trains middle, highschool, and college athletes to be role models to other students in addressing gender violence (Katz et al. 2011). GreenDot, a bystander focused power-based violence prevention program trains students, faculty, and staff in high schools and colleges who are leaders of different sub-communities on college campuses (Coker et al. 2011, 2014; Cook-Craig et al. 2014). Cares (2013) described how on college campuses faculty can play an important role in discussions about violence and victimization. Other key change agents are those 15 % of individuals in a community who are willing to be "innovators or early adopters" of a new message (Rogers 2002). These are the people who connect more quickly to the new message and behaviors, try them out and can be catalysts for the perception by others that this is a good idea that is catching on. This research suggests that if a community has limited prevention resources, a focus on key leaders and early adopters may create more change than small doses of prevention across larger numbers of people. It would be interesting to conduct research comparing communities who put resources into more focused but intensive training of key leaders to those that start by trying to reach everyone.

5.2.2 Changing Norms

The most well discussed avenue of peer influence in the prevention literature is via social pressure in the form of norms. Research finds links not only between peer norms and use of violence but between attitudes toward SV prevention and perceptions of what peers think (Berkowitz 2005; Brown 2006; Paul and Gray 2011; Stein 2007; Strang and Peterson 2013; Zimbardo and Leippe 1991 for reviews). One college student put it this way, "Seeing other people around you doing it. If you see someone else help someone, you're all of a sudden thinking, oh man, I should have helped that person before them, or, I wanna help someone too because I forgot how good it is to do that sort of thing."

5.2.2.1 Universal Helping Norms That May Encourage Bystander Action

What norms may be operating to influence bystander behavior? A number of universal norms are relevant to promoting bystander action. Brown (2006) summarized research on the universal "norm of reciprocity" by which we feel obligated to reciprocate if someone has helped us or done something for us. This norm may be activated when bystanders are in a position to help people they know, helping them feel a heightened sense of responsibility for stepping in (Bennett et al. 2014; Maner and Gailliot 2007; McGuire 2003). One way to motivate bystanders may be to remind them that helping friends may make it more likely that they in turn will be helped.

Researchers have described a number of motives for following social norms to bring our attitudes and behaviors in line with others. We have a strong desire to be liked by others and thus seek to fit in, in part by adopting what we think others are thinking and doing (termed "normative influence" p. 280). We also often have ways that we see ourselves and may adopt thought patterns or behaviors that we think go along with that image ("identity influence," Brown 2006). As one student on a college campus remarked, "In terms of helping people like helping people who are subjects to like sexual harassment stuff I think there's social pressure not to tend to help people like that." All of these motives are operating in prevention workshops. If we are to catalyze bystander action we need to connect with people's desire to know what to do by conveying actions that are expected. We also need to be sensitive to people's desire to be liked and the barriers bystander behavior may present if an individual tries an action and is rejected by those they try to help or by other bystanders.

It may be useful to research and test out how different bystander prevention settings may help to change norms. For example, prevention work often happens in convenience settings such as classrooms or presentations on campus that individuals can choose to attend separately from people they know. The norms described above suggest that training bystanders in SV and IPV may be more effective in settings where universal norms of reciprocity and normative influence are active such as in living groups on college campuses, or athletic teams, spiritual communities, or collections of colleagues in a workplace—locations where individuals already have a relationships (Gidycz et al. 2011; Miller et al. 2012b). Further, perhaps in addition to making public commitments to being active bystanders themselves, we should also ask people to publically pledge to support others when others take action. Bystanders need to support other bystanders. Such efforts have the potential to change norms about supporting bystander action when others do it, changing the community context and reducing cues in the environment that inhibit bystanders' actions out of concerns about being judged negatively.

Finally, we may want to do more to leverage "identity influence" by starting prevention work in communities with assessments of what community members value and how they see themselves. We can then create pro-bystander messages that fit with those identities. For example, descriptions of social marketing campaigns for the U.S. military connect bystander messages to identities of strength and teamwork (Potter and Stapleton 2012). Norms researchers also find that social norms influence attitudes and behaviors only to the extent that individuals identify with the people they are being asked to compare themselves to, they need to see themselves as part of the social norms reference group (Wenzel 2004). Thus, finding ways to make bystander norms locally specific and relevant may enhance their effects. At the University of Richmond and the University of Texas at Austin they named bystander training and campaigns after school mascots.

5.2.2.2 Changing Violence Specific Social Norms in the Community

While leveraging universal norms may help promote bystander action, addressing IPV and SV specific norms in the community is also necessary. Norms about whether coercion is okay to use in relationships, norms about whether it is acceptable to help or even to discuss IPV and SV publically, norms about whether to support other bystanders who take action to interrupt risky situations, norms about whether and when it is okay to interfere when someone is making sexual advances toward someone else or when someone is being controlling of their partner, norms about what types of bystander action are socially sanctioned. For example, a study in Spain found low levels of discussion about IPV and low levels of trust that authorities would respond to it (Gracia and Herrero 2006). Most participants who witnessed IPV did not report it to police.

Norms are part of the framework of how institutions and communities operate (Raymond et al. 2014). We need to find ways to make these norms more explicit and visible so that they can be examined, discussed, challenged and replaced. Researchers noted success in doing this even with complicated community problems and embedded cultural norms like sexism (Becker and Swim 2011; Raymond et al. 2014). Norms can then be either shifted or replaced entirely through processes of "normative reframing" or "normative innovation" (Raymond et al. 2014, p. 197). For example, researchers describe how internationally the problems of sexual assault and domestic violence were for many years not framed as problems but as part of family or relationship processes. Decades of activism created a new term "violence against women" and replaced cultural norms of male privilege around sexual behavior and power in relationships with the idea that these acts are crimes and violations of women's basic human rights. This opened the door to policies for bringing perpetrators to justice and resouces for victims. Bystander intervention is now a next step in this norms change process which can help people see IPV and SV not as individual problems but as community problems that everyone has a responsibility to address.

Changing norms requires introduction of reframed or new norms through initial persuasion techniques and then later through promoting imitation and widespread dissemination (Rogers et al. 2014). Paul and Gray (2011) described two different types of social norms that are important to understand for prevention. Injunctive norms are about behavior that is expected and they are important in initial attempts to change communities through new messages about what was approved behavior. Descriptive norms describe what people actually do and can be used later in prevention as models of behaviors we want people to imitate. Research showed that in environments with injunctive and behavioral norms that do not discourage interpersonal violence, students were less likely to be defenders or prosocial bystanders and in community contexts residents perceived fewer reasons to justify neighbors getting involved to help relationship violence victims (McDonnell et al. 2011; Ruggieria et al. 2013; Sapouna 2010). On the other hand injunctive norms in support of bystander action have been related to greater self-reported behaviors and perceptions that others are taking greater action (Brown et al., in press; McDonnell et al. 2011). Social marketing campaign approaches such as the Red Flag campaign in Virginia or Know Your Power™ (Potter 2012) are examples of interventions that focus on SV and IPV. They aim to change descriptive and injunctive norms by modeling what bystanders should do and show local community members demonstrating the behavior. Indeed, social norms researchers have often highlighted the utility of using posters, stories in the media and other community level techniques for getting new messages out (Haines 1996; Glider et al. 2001). Social marketing campaigns have been associated with improved awareness and sense of responsibility for taking action against sexual and relationship violence (Potter 2012) and decreased rates of victimization (Taylor et al. 2013). Indeed, the best evaluated teen dating violence prevention program includes a component where participants create a poster campaign and theater performance for their school (Foshee et al. 2014).

Part of changing norms is also diffusing the new or reframed norms. Modeling by leaders who are looked up to as having informational or normative influence are a piece of this change strategy. For example, Kelly described changing safe sex and risk reduction practices for HIV prevention by using popular opinion leaders (Kelly 2004). In the violence field, new programs that get parents to talk with their children about alcohol and sexual assault before they head to college showed some effectiveness (Testa et al. 2010) as are programs for young athletes that are delivered by their coaches (Miller et al. 2012b). What this suggests is that a foundation of bystander prevention work to end SV and IPV should start by training key leaders at all levels of the community as active bystanders—not just high profile athletes on campus or just students in middle, highschool or college. Bystander training is needed for faculty, teachers, administrators (Cares 2013) and outside of college campuses, it is needed by spiritual and community leaders and parents of children of all ages. Simply encouraging more public discussions of SV and IPV may be helpful as community members who report more public discussions also report more positive views of bystander actions such as reporting IPV to police (Gracia and Herrero 2006).

5.2.2.3 The Problem of Misperceiving Norms

There can also be problems with how individuals interpret or perceive norms so that they think others are doing or approving of bystander action less than people actually are. These misperceptions suppress bystander intent and action (Fabiano et al. 2003; Paul and Gray 2011). The good news is that perceptions of norms can be changed (Gidycz et al. 2011) by exposing individuals to new descriptive and injunctive norms (Haines 1996; Haines and Barker 2003; Paul and Gray 2011; Perkins et al. 2011). That is, it is helpful to present correct information about what people actually do or expect. Most people do not abuse their partner, most students have intervened to help someone related to sexual assault when given the opportunity to do so, most people disapprove of the use of violence in relationships and most people are supportive of bystander intervention (Brown et al.,

5.2 Changing Action Coil 2: Contextual Processes   93

in press; McMahon et al. 2015; Paul and Gray 2011). For example, educational workshops for men to correct perceptions that peers are unsupportive of bystander action, that peers support the use of coercion in relationships, or that peers are disengaged from prevention efforts have shown promising results (Fabiano et al. 2003; Gidycz et al. 2011; Stein 2007). These strategies and the ones in the section above are a version of Wilson's (2011) "story prompting." This prevention strategy, discussed more below, nudges people toward new ways of seeing themselves and their place in their community. These new lenses may make it more likely that people attend to information consistent with these new narratives (that I am a helpful bystander, that I am someone who cares about respect and equality in relationships). Equipped with new narratives, people change their behavior in healthy and prosocial ways. We need to do more to develop tools to assess norms related to SV and IPV in different communities and use these tools as key parts of community needs assessments conducted before we design our prevention strategies. Campus climate surveys have been highlighted recently as a tool for informing improved prevention and response efforts for SV and IPV (White House Task Force to Protect Students from Sexual Assault 2014, notalone.gov). Measuring norms should be a component of these surveys and broadcasting descriptive norms results should follow. Prevention work should discuss community norms that are active as well as misperceptions of norms in addition to more traditional knowledge building presentations (Banyard 2014).

5.2.2.4 Internalizing New Norms and Changing Bystander Identity

It is important to link these larger social norms to internalized personal norms (Wenzel 2004). While research on social norms attends to what we need to change in the community to create more helpful bystander action, there are also processes we need to encourage within the individual. One way to do this is to use narrative techniques which Wilson (2011) describes as "story-editing" and "story-prompting" (p. 11). He asserts that part of how we change behavior is to help people see themselves differently, to see themselves as individuals who do not tolerate interpersonal violence and take action to address it. He reviews a growing literature on the use of writing about both negative and positive events and how expressive writing allows people to make sense of an event and see it in a new way. For example, one set of researchers were able to change women's endorsement of sexist beliefs by having them complete daily diaries where they indicated how many of a list of obvious and more subtle sexist interactions they experienced or witnessed each day (Becker and Swim 2011). Making these incidents more obvious changed beliefs. For men, the intervention needed to take the story further. Reductions in sexist attitudes occurred when men completed the checklist but also reflected and wrote about the emotional impact of the sexist behaviors, using the diaries to not only increase awareness but empathy. This narrative technique could be used in bystander training. In between training sessions bystanders could be asked to keep daily diaries of incidents of risk they observed along the full continuum of SV and IPV including comments and harassing gestures. Participants, particularly men, would also be asked to reflect and indicate what negative emotions they thought the victim experienced or they experienced themselves. Similar narrative tracking could be done of observed bystander actions.

Wilson asserts that it is also possible to give people a new story, to push them in the right direction through "story-prompting" which are stimuli which help people to think about things in a different way as modeled by others. Recently, we see bystanders mentioned more often in news stories about sexual and relationship violence. However, all too often this is only in the context of pointing out how they have not helped. Using Wilson's model, what if we developed local community videos of positive bystander stories or narratives of bystanders who overcame barriers to find successful and safe ways to take action? This would help potential bystanders "re-story" (Wilson 2011, p. 11) how sexual and relationship violence unfold, to add in helpful bystanders who prevent negative consequences. This storying approach could be used in communities over time, encouraging bystanders to write about and reflect on how they tried to help and how it worked or could have gone better. Over time communities would weave together more empowered narratives about taking positive actions. Role plays, video games, or virtual reality might also provide such opportunities for individuals to take on different stories about their role and success as bystanders (Jouriles et al. 2014). These individual stories also then have the potential to become cultural stories of helping and provide data about descriptive norms that can help communities and the individuals within them be more likely to label themselves and their neighbors as "helpful" or as defenders, supporters, spokespeople.

5.2.3 Policy Change Can Impact Individual Action

Another component of action coil two is policies that impact bystander action. Mossholder et al. (2011) discussed how different human resources contexts (that consist of norms but also policies) in organizations impacted helping among employees. Indeed, we know that norms change needs to be leveraged not only through internal motivation (as with storying approaches described above) but also through external motivations (Raymond et al. 2014). In prevention, research is clear that efforts that extend into the community and are more comprehensive and far reaching have more of an impact on changing behaviors and attitudes (Wandersman and Florin 2003). Policies help to create the reward and consequence structures in which bystanders make choices about taking action. They also shape the presence or absence of different risk and protective factors.

One piece of policy change involves external rewards and consequences for a behavior (Zimbardo and Leippe 1991 for a review). SV and IPV policies can make a difference. Miller et al. (2012a) found that participants' asked to read vignettes about a sexual assault assigned more blame to victims if given instructions that the law about sexual assault was unclear, compared to participants who were told the law was clear. Strang and Peterson (2013) found less verbal coercion among men who perceived greater certainty that punishment would be associated with their behavior. Maimon et al. (2012) found less school violence among some particularly at-risk youth in schools with more severe sanctions for violence. Paul and Grey (2011) discussed how changing negative sanctions for interpersonal violence and enforcing them will lead to perceptions of costs of violence as being greater than the benefits gained by exercising power in this way. It may also make clear to bystanders that taking action is appropriate and expected. What is more, clear policies about SV and IPV will better mobilize professional helpers like law enforcement, who bystanders may need to call to intervene. Some policies are specific to bystanders. Several states have laws that you must help someone in "danger of physical harm" (Vermont Statutes) or call 911 if you witness a sexual assault (Rhode Island General Laws). These laws are designed to increase bystander responsibility and action.

But how do we create these policy changes? An interesting strategy called "safety audits" has been used to carefully examine policies and organizational procedures in relation to how they support or work against IPV victims' safety (Pence and McMahon 2003; Sadusky et al. 2010). Similar audits could be done of policies and practices related to sexual and relationship violence and how they may directly or indirectly support or work against bystander and prevention work. For example, the coding in an audit could ask how different school policies encourage or discourage bystander action? Earlier in this book I discussed research that showed that college students often chose not to step into help in situations of sexual or relationship violence because of school alcohol policies under which they themselves may have gotten in trouble or gotten a victim in trouble for underage drinking if they called formal helpers. In this situation, a bystander audit might reveal the need for Good Samaritan policies to protect students who are reporting a problem. One student remarked, "Knowing some sort of Good-Samaritan act or law—knowing that it can't come back up on them if they try to help someone… really does a lot of good." Further, a recent news story from Canada described St. Mary's College which had clear policies against sexual assault and yet included a tradition of student leaders teaching chants that condoned sexual contact without consent (Kingkade 2013). An audit of a school's tradition, website language, etc. could be a good place to start to examine how messages, norms and policies may be working against strong violence prevention messages and dissuade bystanders from acting (Hayes-Smith and Hayes-Smith 2009).

Policies can also change the presence of risk and protective factors for violence and for helping. For example, Taylor et al. (2013) found that for reducing gender violence in schools the more effective strategy was not individual focused classroom curricula but identifying "hotspots" for violence and increasing staff presence there at risky times combined with school policy changes related to consequences for gender based violence. Campuses and communities alike have long been working on environmental change related to alcohol use. Research found that reducing the number of liquor outlets or making changes to bar hours or creating substance-free residence halls on campuses could reduce problem drinking but also sexual assaults (Lippy and DeGue 2014; Scribner et al. 2010, 2011).

Finally, policies affect resource allocation. We need to change how we think about and do prevention by integrating it more into the fabric of what schools, communities, and college campuses do; not just as an add on but an integral part of an organization or school's mission. We see the seeds of this in social emotional learning curricula (Durlak et al. 2011) for younger children which combines academics with lessons to promote positive relationships, coping, and self regulation. This sort of broad approach has not been yet been widely integrated in workplaces, in high schools or on college campuses. For instance, might it be possible to have a required prevention core curriculum in addition to an academic core curriculum across four years at college? Can bystander training become part of workplace professional development requirements? An environment in which prevention conversations occupy a more central place would be places where bystanders could receive ongoing support and feedback rather than one time training sessions. Prevention is too often a voluntary extra activity rather than something that is important enough to be mandatory.

5.3 Changing Action Coil 3: Influencing the Event Itself

What happens during the actual event that a bystander witnesses is a third action coil. As described in Chap. 4, key components of this coil include the scripts or plan of action that a person has in place for helping. In Chap. 4 I discussed how there may be a mismatch between scripts that individuals have for general helping, and what they may need to do to take action in instances of sexual and relationship violence. This disconnect is due in part to the complexity of sexual and relationship violence but may also be due to the variety of roles that a bystander can potentially play as the situation unfolds. I consider change mechanisms related to each of these components of the event action coil below.

5.3.1 Social Scripts

Our interactions with others are governed by social scripts (Brown 2006). They help us know what to expect and can provide shortcuts for knowing how to act in different situations. However, we get anxious when we encounter situations that we do not have scripts for, or where our usual scripts do not fit (Avery et al. 2009). Prevention tools need to give potential bystanders new helping scripts to reduce anxiety and uncertainty that may be generated when they encounter sexual violence or relationship abuse risk. Indeed one study found adolescents' scores on a measure of intergroup anxiety was related to lower intent to take action against racial bullying (Abbott and Cameron 2014). Avery et al. (2009) described "scripting" as an intervention to promote successful interracial interactions. Scripting consists of planned opportunities for structured dialogues that give individuals practice with specific behavioral instructions. Many bystander education programs provide opportunities for role play discussions (Mentors in Violence Prevention; Katz et al. 2011). However, these are often not specifically scripted with a series of steps a bystander should take. Perhaps such role plays should include more detail, or a step by step set of behaviors and questions or conversations starters, at least at first. Individuals could then practice a structured script about intervening before then being given more open ended scenarios where they can create their own responses.

Some of these scripts form the basis of online training programs, where individuals watch a scenario unfold on their screen (Schewe 2013) or interactive theater where a script is acted out on stage. Social marketing campaigns like Know Your Power™ show people specific examples of what they can do and use visual images in which people can see themselves (Potter et al. 2011). In Bringing in the Bystander™, participants create their own specific bystander plan—a new script for what they might do. Next steps are also needed to give individuals direct practice with these scripts. Further, individuals may need a chance to loop back after trying scripts in the real world. How did they work? How might they need to be changed? Thus, creating change in the event action coil is directly connected to the outcome action coil discussed in more detail below. Future research should examine the impact of prevention strategies on helping scripts.

As noted above, new knowledge needs to be connected to what people already know and find important. Thus, work to develop new scripts for bystanders needs to be grounded in their lived experience and an awareness of the different roles bystanders can play. These different roles (defender, supporter, dissenter, spokesperson) may need different scripts. In much of the bystander literature, bystanders to sexual and relationship abuse are thought of as almost exclusively as direct defenders of victims. A separate literature on disclosure considers them as supporters of victims. We need to do more in our prevention work to consider these and other roles together. We need to do more in our research to examine different correlates and outcomes of these roles and to put training experiences on these different issues in one integrated set of strategies.

5.4 Changing Action Coil 4: Influencing Outcomes

The final coil in the model proposed in Chap. 4 describes outcomes of helping. When considering this coil we can ask what strategies are needed to make positive outcomes more likely and to guard against retaliation against bystanders, bystanders being hurt or other unintended consequences of bystander focused prevention. Change needs to focus on keeping bystanders safe and increasing the chances that bystander action will help victims. A number of strategies are needed. The first is more research. As stated earlier we know relatively little about consequences of actions taken by bystanders to prevent SV and IPV. We need research studies that answer questions about what actions carry few negative consequences for bystanders and what types of strategies are most helpful for diffusing or changing a risky situation.

5.4.1 Action Effectiveness

Greater understanding of what actions are effective under what conditions will enable the design of prevention strategies to more specifically help bystanders choose their actions. Current bystander efforts do focus on expanding bystanders' toolkits for helping so that they have a variety of options that can be used. Bystanders also need opportunities to practice these new options through role plays so that techniques are more readily available in the stress of a bystander action moment. Interesting recent work from the field of communication offers a paradigm for researching answers to what actions are most effective, "message design logic" (White and Malkowski 2014). This model puts together an individual's implicit ideas about how to use communication to influence a situation with a person's goals for that situation and the strategies they choose to reach their goals. There are three patterns of logic described that frame how individuals develop their communications. Some individuals used "expressive logic" to "express thoughts and feelings, a more simple logic that relies on conveying information (White and Malkowski 2014, p. 95)." Others used more sophisticated "rhetorical logic" which "reflects an understanding of communication as creating an opportunity to negotiate (p. 95)" to create the outcomes you want to see happen. A third group uses more "conventional" logic which focuses on following social rules and pointing out consequences of not following them. Past research in other communication situations showed that expressive logic may be less effective than rhetorical logic. It has been applied to understand how bystanders intervened in hypothetical drinking situations. In one study, participants read a vignette where a young man and woman at a college party were drinking and the young man made sexual advances that seemed unwelcome. They asked participants what their goals would be as bystanders and what they would say if they were in the situation. A measure of general beliefs about communication was also administered. Key goals expressed included safety, trying to get the young man to leave the woman alone, making sure the young woman was not isolated with the young man, and trying to figure out what the young woman wanted in the situation. The researchers found that for some goals there was a clear link between the action strategy chosen and the expressed goal while for other goals there was not. For example, if participants said their goal was to separate the couple then participants were more likely to say they would try to ask questions or enter the conversation with the couple. On the other hand, when the expressed goal was safety participants tended to equally report using various strategies of asking questions, entering the conversation or warning about the riskiness of the situation (e.g. telling the young man that the woman was too drunk to consent). The researchers hypothesized that more logical matching between goals and strategies would make the communication more effective. What was also interesting was that beliefs about communication were related to choice of strategy. Individuals in the "expressive logic" category focused on warning the young man. Those in the "rhetorical" category more often described inserting themselves into the conversation or asking questions to learn more about what the young woman wanted. This research paradigm could be used to test the consequences of different bystander actions for influencing different SV and IPV situations and the effectiveness of different communication beliefs. Research should examine whether expressive versus rhetorical styles are more or less helpful in SV and IPV bystander situations, or to what extent goal to strategy matching improves bystander effectiveness. If the results show patterns of effectiveness, these research activities could be incorporated into prevention programs to help potential bystanders assess their preferred communication logic patterns (expressive, rhetorical, conventional) as well as make more transparent what they see as their goals as bystanders in different situations. Such reflection could provide chances for bystanders to more carefully consider how to best match strategies to goals in the situation, but also how to practice more complex communication patterns that might achieve more success in the complex interactions of SV and IPV prevention.

5.4.2 Building Collective Efficacy

A second strategy for action coil four is building collective efficacy. Research is clear that collective efficacy is related to violence prevention and reduction and to bystander action (Edwards et al. 2014). Several articles have presented case studies of how community engagement was used to prevent violence by getting people involved, making them aware of local data about a problem and leveraging policy and program changes in the community (Beck et al. 2012; Bowen et al. 2004). From the perspective of bystanders, communities with greater efficacy may be more supportive of their actions and create a lower likelihood of retaliation. Collective efficacy may also make it easier for people to take action together. We need more research and descriptions of what specific strategies are useful for actually building collective efficacy in a community. One set of researchers noted the importance of (1) raising awareness about the importance of collective efficacy and its benefits (2) engaging in community development by bringing in opportunities and resources for community members and leaders to build skills and capacity for building collective efficacy, (3) creating opportunities for community members to work on common goals including that meetings be about not just working on tasks but also about building relationships and getting to know one another in the community (Beck et al. 2012). Community coalitions or collaboratives of different leaders and members are a facet of this work (Pennington-Zoelner 2009), and a facet that has been studied on its own and found effective in improving physical health indicators in communities across a number of studies (see Roussos and Fawcett 2000 for a review). Communities need to build spaces for people who are potential formal and informal helpers to come together and work together on more collaborative bystander action.

5.4.3 Training Professional Responders

A third change strategy focuses on training professional responders to assess the roles of bystanders and finding safe ways for bystanders to reach out for help. This is particularly true in relation to the social position of bystanders. We need to make sure that stereotypes and biases against individuals from underrepresented groups (whether racial minorities or sexual minorities) do not lead to erroneous perceptions of who is the perpetrator and who is the active bystander in a situation nor to ignoring or minimizing the severity of the situation or to victims getting in trouble for secondary behavior like underage drinking when bystanders intervene. Further, formal helpers need to continue to build trust in communities of potential bystanders so that formal helpers will be seen as a resource. This is particularly important when bystanders are needed as witnesses or when bystanders need help protecting their own safety.

Related to this, hotlines in communities are often perceived as for victims only rather than for bystanders and they are often siloed by issue (with different numbers to call for child maltreatment, domestic violence, etc.). New social marketing campaigns in several communities are providing more general hotlines focused on bystanders. In Colorado, a new program called "Safe2Tell" provides an anonymous community hotline that anyone can use to report someone being hurt. The "Where's the Line?" campaign in Ohio is designed to encourage family and community members to report domestic violence and also includes a new anonymous hotline for bystanders (Seman 2015). This sort of reporting system may make it easier for bystanders to act, especially if they fear retaliation for being identified. It also provides a safe option for involving formal helpers rather than bystanders feeling like they have to intervene directly themselves. This may be particularly important in communities where individuals may be willing to be in the role of a defender but lesswilling to be a witness.

5.4.4 Bystanders Supporting Bystanders

Not only professional responders need training and improvement in responding to bystanders in situations of risk for SV and IPV. We also need to do more to get people to help each other by supporting other bystanders. We need to use strategies like narratives and role playing and perhaps even cooperative online training and games to encourage individuals to see themselves as supporters of other people who help. We need community norms that praise active bystanders and reward them. Communities mobilized in this way will likely present more chances for bystanders to enlist others to help them directly, a safer option in many instances, but will also work against negative consequences for bystanders such as retaliation, loss of friendships, etc.

5.4.5 Safety Nets for Bystanders

Communities must build safety nets and supports for active bystanders. Good Samaritan policies are one way to do this. Campus policies like the "sexual assault amnesty" policy at Elizabeth City State University in North Carolina has a provision for students who call campus authorities to aid someone who has been sexually assaulted. They will not be charged even if they are in violation of the school's alcohol policies (http://www.ecsu.edu/legal/docs/policymanual/Sect.900/900-4-1-5.pdf).

It is also important to create places for bystanders to come together to debrief and seek support. We cannot simply train bystanders once and have that be the end of it. If bystander intervention is truly a process then training engagement with bystanders needs to persist over time. Our prevention strategies need to be coils not brief one time events. Addressing the topic of bystander action across the lifespan in a more intentional and direct manner will not only help individuals build a strong foundation of flexible helping scripts for addressing interpersonal violence but will promote a supportive community context in which retaliation against bystanders and negative responses to helping will be minimized.

5.5 Summary

- Bystander attitude and behavior change has centered mostly on action coil 1 to date and theories of change at this level focus on raising awareness through convincing and persuasive messages that are repeated over time and activities that get potential bystanders to start practicing actions they can take.
- Attention to the broader context of bystander action in action coil two requires prevention strategies that change social norms at peer and community levels as well as the translation of these to new personal norms through narrative strategies.
- Action coil three can be addressed with prevention strategies that go beyond passive messages and presentations to role plays and interactive discussions.
- Action coil four requires community building through policy change, relationship mobilization, and the creation of IPV and SV response systems that bystanders can use with minimal perceived consequences.
- Prevention itself needs to be coils of strategies over time to help bystanders tolerate the complexity of the situations they will encounter, be flexible and creative in their responses, to build tenacity for action processes over time, and to help bystanders better support one another.

5.6 Practice Implications

In this chapter my aim was to look at sexual and relationship violence prevention by mobilizing bystanders from a different angle, the angle of change. It is not enough just to understand what variables make being an active bystander more likely. We also want to change many people's behavior so that they in fact become more active and safe bystanders, so that the action coils described in chapter four become prevention springs. Creating behavior change to activate these springs in communities must be an ongoing process. We need many different prevention messages and tools to meet different people where they are in terms of existing attitudes and motivation. We need messages that motivate and facilitate getting everyone and all communities to move through next steps along the path to ending violence.

While the ultimate goal of prevention is behavior change, many of the correlates of bystander action are attitudes. There are many pathways to attitude change across the social-ecological model, including exposing individuals to new social norms, pointing out inconsistencies between what individuals say they believe and how they have acted, building emotional connections to victims and empathy, and helping individuals see personal relevance in the problem. People also need something new to do and action creates change. They need lessons and practice in new skills for relationship building, conflict resolution, and helping. Thus, our prevention efforts to increase bystander action need to draw from all of these strategies.

A key aspect of examining behavior change is appreciating individual and community differences. Research suggests that while emotional arguments may work for issues that are familiar and of low importance, important and unfamiliar messages like those likely associated with SV and IPV prevention may require more rational arguments and conditions that support this careful thinking (Zimbardo and Leippe 1991). People vary in how much they think about new information and messages depending on how personally relevant they think it is or how distracted they are by other things. As Potter and Stapleton (2011) describe, we need to be flexible in our prevention design, adapting tools from one community to another so that participants see the information as relevant and connected to their experiences.

People, whether individually or collectively as a community, start at different places in terms of awareness, knowledge, and skill sets when they engage with prevention efforts. Not all participants will get there with the same prevention program or even in the same timeframe. Conceptualizing our work as a progression of efforts that incorporate the strategies discussed in this chapter may help us get to better prevention outcomes.

What is important to note is that prevention programs focused on bystander intervention focus mainly on how to create change in bystanders. To that end this chapter summarized change mechanisms with potential bystanders as the recipients of these strategies. However, an equally important and largely unasked question is what change action strategies can bystanders use most effectively and safely to intervene and change the behaviors of friends and acquaintances to promote more positive social norms against violence, in favor of helping, and in support of respectful relationships. Many of the change principles in this chapter may be relevant to finding these answers. More research on bystander consequences and safety will help us learn which change strategies we may best recommend and incorporate into skill building exercises as part of prevention tools.

References

Abbott, N., & Cameron, L. (2014). What makes a young assertive bystander? The effect of intergroup contact, empathy, cultural openness, and in-group bias on assertive bystander intervention intentions. *Journal of Social Issues, 70*, 167–182.

Abraham, C., & Sheeran, P. (2005). The health belief model. In M. Connor & P. Norman (Eds.), *Predicting health behavior* (pp. 28–80). Berkshire, England: Open University Press McGraw Hill.

Ahrens, C. E., Rich, M. D., & Ullman, J. B. (2011). Rehearsing for real life: The impact of the InterACT sexual assault prevention program on self-reported likelihood of engaging in bystander interventions. *Violence Against Women, 17*, 760–776.

Ajzen, I. (1991). The theory of planned behavior. *Organizational Behavior and Human Decision Processes, 50*, 179–211.

Avery, D. R., Richeson, J. A., Hebl, M. R., & Ambady, N. (2009). It does not have to be uncomfortable: The role of behavioral scripts in black–white interracial interactions. *Journal of Applied Psychology, 94*, 1382–1393.

Banyard, V. L. (2008). Measurement and correlates of pro-social bystander behavior: The case of interpersonal violence. *Violence and Victims, 23*, 83–97.

Banyard, V. (2014). Improving college campus based prevention of violence against women: A strategic plan for research built on multi-pronged practices and policies trauma. *Trauma, Violence, and Abuse, 15*, 339–351.

Banyard, V. L., Eckstein, R., & Moynihan, M. M. (2010). Sexual violence prevention: The role of stages of change. *Journal of Interpersonal Violence, 25*, 111–135.

Banyard, V. L., & Moynihan, M. M. (2011). Variation in bystander behavior related to sexual and intimate partner violence prevention: Correlates in a sample of college students. *Psychology of Violence, 1*, 287–301.

Banyard, V. L., Moynihan, M. M., Cares, A. C., & Warner, R. (2014). How do we know if it works? Measuring outcomes in bystander-focused abuse prevention on campuses. *Psychology of Violence, 4*, 101–115.

Banyard, V. L., Potter, S. J., Cares, A., Williams, L. M., Moynihan, M. M., & Stapleton, J. G. (under review). *Ending sexual violence on campuses by improving bystander intervention: Multiple prevention tools working together.*

Banyard, V., Weber, M., Grych, J., & Hamby, S. (in press). Where are the helpful bystanders? Ecological niche and victims' perceptions of bystander intervention. *Journal of Community Psychology.*

Beck, E., Ohmer, M., & Warner, B. (2012). Strategies for preventing neighborhood violence: Toward bringing collective efficacy into social work practice. *Journal of Community Practice, 20*, 225–240.

Becker, J., & Swim, J. K. (2011). Seeing the unseen: Attention to daily encounters as a way to reduce sexist beliefs. *Psychology of Women Quarterly, 35*, 227–242.

Bennett, S., Banyard, V., & Edwards, K. (in preparation). Does who you know matter?: The effect of the relationship between the bystander and the victim and the perpetrator on intent to help in situations involving sexual violence.

Bennett, S., Banyard, V. L., & Garnhart, L. (2014). To act or not to act, that is the question?: Barriers and facilitators of bystander intervention. *Journal of Interpersonal Violence, 29*, 476–496.

Berkowitz, A. D. (2005). An overview of the social norms approach. In L. C. Lederman & L. P. Stewart (Eds.), *Changing the culture of college drinking: A socially situated health communication campaign* (pp. 193–214). Cresskill, N.J.: Hampton Press.

Boher, G., & Dickel, N. (2011). Attitudes and attitude change. *Annual Review of Psychology, 62*, 391–417.

Borges, A., Banyard, V. L., & Moynihan, M. M. (2008). Clarifying consent: Primary prevention of sexual assault on a college campus. *Journal of Prevention and Intervention in the Community, 36*, 75–88.

Bowen, L. K., Gwiasda, V., & Brown, M. M. (2004). Engaging community residents to prevent violence. *Journal of Interpersonal Violence, 19*, 356–367.

Brown, J. D. (2006). *Social psychology*. Boston: McGraw Hill.

Bushman, B. J., & Anderson, C. A. (2009). Comfortably numb desensitizing effects of violent media on helping others. *Psychological Science, 20*, 273–277.

Cares, A. C. (2013). *What is the role of college faculty in stopping sexual assault? The Resource: Newsletter of the National Sexual Violence Resource Center, Spring Summer, 16–30*. Enola, PA: NSVRC.

Carpenter, S. K., Cepeda, N. J., Rohrer, D., Kang, S. H. K., & Pashler, H. (2012). Using spacing to enhance diverse forms of learning: Review of recent research and implications for instruction. *Educational Psychology Review, 24*, 369–378.

Chaudoir, S. R., & Fisher, J. D. (2010). The disclosure process model: Understanding disclosure decision making and postdisclosure outcomes among people living with a concealable stigmatized identity. *Psychological Bulletin, 136*, 236–256.

Cimini, M. D., Rivero, E. M., Bernier, J. E., Stanley, J. A., Murray, A. D., Anderson, D. A., et al. (2014). Implementing an audience-speific small-group gatekeeper training program to respond to suicide risk among college students: A case study. *Journal of American College Health, 62*, 92–100.

Coker, A. L., Cook-Craig, P. G., Williams, C. M., Fisher, B. S., Clear, E. R., Garcia, L. S., & Hegge, L. M. (2011). Evaluation of green dot: An active bystander intervention to reduce sexual violence on college campuses. *Violence Against Women, 17*, 777–796.

Coker, A. L., Fisher, B. S., Bush, H. M., Swan, S. C., Williams, C. M., Clear, E. R., & DeGue, S. (2014). Evaluation of the green dot bystander intervention to reduce interpersonal violence among college students across three campuses. *Violence Against Women, 20*, 1179–1202.

Cook-Craig, P. G., Coker, A. L., Clear, E. R., Garcia, L. S., Bush, H. M., Brancato, C. J., et al. (2014). Challenge and opportunity in evaluating a diffusion-based active bystanding prevention program green dot in high schools. *Violence Against Women, 20*, 1179–1202.

Cox, P. J., Lang, K. S., Townsend, S. M., & Campbell, R. (2010). The rape prevention and education (RPE) theory model of community change: Connecting individual and social change. *Journal of Family Social Work, 13*, 297–312.

Crisp, R. J., & Turner, R. N. (2012). The imagined contact hypothesis. In J. Olson & M. P. Zanna (Eds.), *Advances in experimental social psychology* (Vol. l46, pp. 125–182). Orlando: Academic Press.

Das, M, Bosh, S., Miller, E., O'Conner, B., & Verma, R. (2012). *Engaging coaches and athletes in fostering gender equity: Findings from the Parivartan program in Mumbai, India*. Summary report. New Delhi, India, International Center for Research on Women [ICRW], May 2012. http://www.popline.org/node/561549#sthash.xyvwa5DO.dpuf

DeGue, S., Valle, A., Holt, M. K., Massetti, G. M., Matjasko, J. L., & Tharp, A. T. (2014). A systematic review of primary prevention strategies for sexual violence perpetration. *Aggression and Violent Behavior, 19*, 346–362.

Durlak, J. A., Weissberg, R. P., Dymnicki, A. B., Taylor, R. D., & Schellinger, K. B. (2011). The impact of enhancing students' social and emotional learning: A meta-analysis of school-based universal interventions. *Child Development, 82*, 405–432.

References

Edwards, K., Banyard, V., Moynihan, M. M., Rodenheiser, K., & Demers, J. (in preparation). Community readiness to engage: Assessing campus efforts to prevent sexual and relationship violence.

Edwards, K., Mattingly, M. J., Dixon. K. J., & Banyard, V. L. (2014). Community matters: Intimate partner violence among young adults. *American Journal of Community Psychology, 53*, 198–207.

Everfi. (2014). Haven (http://www.everfi.com/haven

Every Choice. (2014). http://every-choice.com

Fabiano, P. M., Perkins, H. W., Berkowitz, A., Linkenbach, J., & Stark, C. (2003). Engaging men as social justice allies in ending violence against women: Evidence for a social norms approach. *Journal of American College Health, 52*, 105–112.

Foshee, V. A., McNaughton Reyes, L., Agnew-Brune, C. B., Simon, T. R., Vagi, K. J., Lee, R. D., & Suchindran, C. (2014). *The effects of the evidence-based safe dates dating abuse prevention program on other youth violence outcomes.* Online first: Prevention Science.

Frohmann, L. (2005). The framing safety project: Photographs and narratives by battered women. *Violence Against Women, 11*, 1396–1419.

Gidycz, C. A., Lynn, S. J., Rich, C. L., Marioni, N. L., Loh, C., Blackwell, L. M., et al. (2001). The evaluation of a sexual assault risk reduction program: A multisite investigation. *Journal of Consulting and Clinical Psychology, 69*, 1073–1078.

Gidycz, C. A., Orchowski, L. M., & Berkowitz, A. D. (2011). Preventing sexual aggression among college men: An evaluation of a social norms and bystander intervention program. *Violence Against Women, 17*, 720–742.

Glider, P., Midyett, S. J., Mills-Novoa, B., Johannessen, K., & Collins, C. (2001). Challenging the collegiate rite of passage: A campus-wide social marketing media campaign to reduce binge drinking. *Journal of Drug Education, 31*, 207–220.

Gracia, E., & Herrero, J. (2006). Public attitudes toward reporting partner violence against women and reporting behavior. *Journal of Marriage and Family, 68*, 759–768.

Greitemeyer, T., & Cox, C. (2013). There's no "I" in team: Effects of cooperative video games on cooperative behavior. *European Journal of Social Psychology, 43*, 224–228.

Greitemeyer, T., & Osswald, S. (2010). Effects of prosocial video games on prosocial behavior. *Journal of Personality and Social Psychology, 98*, 211–221.

Greitemeyer, T., Traut-Mattausch, E., & Osswald, S. (2012). How to ameliorate negative effects of violent video games on cooperation: Play it cooperatively in a team. *Computers in Human Behavior, 28*, 1465–1470.

Grimley, D., Prochaska, J. O., Velicer, W. F., Blais, L. M., & DiClemente, C. C. (1994). The transtheoretical model of change. In T. Brimthaupt & R. Lipka (Eds.), *Changing the self: Philosophies, techniques, and experiences* (pp. 201–227). NY: SUNY Press.

Guerette, R. T., Flexon, J. L., & Marquez, C. (2013). Instigating bystander intervention in the prevention of alcohol-impaired driving: Analysis of data regarding mass media campaigns. *Journal of Studies on Alcohol and Drugs, 74*, 205–211.

Haines, M. (1996). *A social norms approach to preventing binge drinking at colleges and universities.* The Higher Education Center for Alcohol and Other Drug Prevention.

Haines, M., & Barker, G. P. (2003). The Northern Illinois University experiment: A longitudinal case study of the social norms approach. In H. W. Perkins (Ed.), *The social norms approach to preventing school and college age substance abuse: A handbook for educators, counselors, and clinicians* (pp. 21–34). San Francisco, CA, US: Jossey-Bass.

Hamby, S., Banyard, V. & Grych, J. (in press). Prevention of interpersonal violence. In *Handbook of Clinical Psychology.*

Hayes-Smith & Hayes-Smith. (2009). A website content analysis of women's resources and sexual assault literature on college campuses. *Critical Criminology, 17*, 109–123.

Heppner, M. J., Good, G. E., Hillenbrand-Gunn, T. L., Hawkins, A. K., Hacquard, L. L., Nichols, R. K., et al. (2001). Examining sex differences in altering attitudes about rape: A test of the Elaboration Likelihood Model. *Journal of Counseling and Development, 73*, 640–647.

Jouriles, E. N., Kleinsasser, A., Rosenfield, D., & McDonald, R. (2014, October 27). Measuring bystander behavior to prevent sexual violence: Moving beyond self reports. *Psychology of Violence*. Advance online publication. http://dx.doi.org/10.1037/a0038230

Katz, J., Heisterkamp, H. A., & Fleming, W. M. (2011). The social justice roots of the Mentors in Violence Prevention model and its application in a high school setting. *Violence Against Women, 17*, 684–702.

Kelly, J. (2004). Popular opinion leaders and HIV prevention peer education: Resolving discrepant findings, and implications for the development of effective community programmes. *AIDS Care, 16*, 139–150.

Kingkade, T. (Sept. 6, 2013). St. Mary's University students' pro-rape chant condemned after 5 years of use. *Huffington Post*. Accessed from http://www.huffingtonpost.com/2013/09/06/st-marys-university-chant-rape_n_3879903.html

Kleinsasser, A., Jouriles, E. N., McDonald, R., & Rosenfield, D. (2015). An online bystander intervention program for the prevention of sexual violence. *Psychology of Violence, 5*(3), 227–235.

Latané, B. & Darley, J. M. (1970). *The unresponsive bystander: Why doesn't he help?* New York, NY: Appleton-Century-Crofts.

Leone, R. M., Parrott, D. J., Swartout, K. M., & Tharp, A. D. (2015). Masculinity and bystander attitudes: Moderating effects of masculine gender role stress. *Psychology of Violence*. (Online first).

Levine, M., & Thompson, K. (2004). Identity, place, and bystander intervention: Social categories and helping after natural disasters. *The Journal of Social Psychology, 144*, 229–245.

Levine, M., Prosser, A., Evans, D., & Reicher, S. (2005). Identity and emergency interventions: How social group membership and inclusiveness of group boundaries shape helping behavior. *Personality and Social Psychology Bulletin, 31*, 443–453.

Lippy, C., & DeGue, S. (2014). Exploring alcohol policy approaches to prevent sexual violence perpetration. *Trauma, Violence, & Abuse*. Online first.

Madden, T. J., Ellen, P. S., & Ajzen, I. (1992). A comparison of the theory of planned behavior and the theory of reasoned action. *Personality and Social Psychology Bulletin, 18*, 3–9.

Maimon, D., Antonaccio, O., & French, M. T. (2012). Severe sanctions easy choice? Investigating the role of school sanctions in preventing adolescent violence offending. *Criminology, 50*, 495–524.

Maner, K. K., & Gailliot, M. T. (2007). Altruism and egoism: Prosocial motivations for helping depend on relationship context. *European Journal of Social Psychology, 37*, 347–358.

McCauley, H. L., Tancredi, D. J., Silverman, J. G., Decker, M. R., Austin, S. B., McCormick, M. C., & Miller, E. (2013). Gender-equitable attitudes, bystander behavior, and recent abuse perpetration against heterosexual dating partners of male high school athletes. *American Journal of Public Health, 103*, 1882–1887.

McDonnell, K. A., Burke, J. G., Gielen, A. C., O'Campo, P., & Weidl, M. (2011). Women's perceptions of their community's social norms towards assisting women who have experienced intimate partner violence. *Journal of Urban Health, 88*, 240–253.

McGuire, A. M. (2003). "It was nothing"—Extending evolutionary models of altruism by two social cognitive biases in judgments of the costs and benefits of helping. *Social Cognition, 21*, 363–394.

McMahon, S., Banyard, V., & McMahon, S. (2015). Incoming college students' bystander behaviors to prevent sexual violence. *Journal of College Student Development, 56*, 488–493

McMahon, S., Postmus, J. L., & Koenick, R. A. (2011). Conceptualizing the engaging bystander approach to sexual violence prevention on college campuses. *Journal of College Student Development, 52*, 115–130.

Miller, A. K., Markman, K. D., Amacker, A. M., & Menaker, T. A. (2012a). Expressed sexual assault legal context and victim culpability attributions. *Journal of Interpersonal Violence, 27*, 1023–1039.

References

Miller, E., Tancredi, D. J., McCauley, H. L., Decker, M. R., Virata, M. C., Anderson, H. A., Stetkevich, N., Brown, E. W., Miodeen, F., & Silverman, J. (2012b). "Coaching boys into men": A cluster-randomized controlled trial of a dating violence prevention program. *Journal of Adolescent Health*.

Mossholder, K. W., Richardson, H. A., & Settoon, R. P. (2011). Human resource systems and helping in organizations: A relational perspective. *Academy of Management Review, 36*, 33–52.

Moynihan, M. M., Banyard, V. L., Cares, A. C., Potter, S. J., Williams, L. M., & Stapleton, J. G. (2015). Encouraging responses in sexual and relationship violence prevention: What program effects remain one year later? *Journal of Interpersonal Violence, 30*, 110–132.

Nation, M., Crusto, C., Wandersman, A., Kumpfer, K. L., Seybolt, D., Morrissey-Kane, E., & Davino, K. (2003). What works in prevention: Principles of effective prevention programs. *American Psychologist, 58*, 449–456.

National Sexual Violence Resource Center. (2014) http://www.nsvrc.org/publications/nsvrc-publications/engaging-bystanders-sexual-violence-prevention

One Love Foundation. (2015). https://www.joinonelove.org/join-the-movement/escalation-workshop/

Paluck, E. L., & Green, D. P. (2009). Prejudice reduction: What works? A review and assessment of research and practice. *Annual Review of Psychology, 60*, 339–367.

Paul, L. A., & Gray, M. J. (2011). Sexual assault programming on college campuses: Using social psychological belief and behavior change principles to improve outcomes. *Trauma, Violence, & Abuse, 12*(2), 99–109.

Pence, E., & McMahon, M. (2003). Working from inside and outside institutions: How safety audits can help courts' decision making around domestic violence and child maltreatment. *Juvenile and Family Court Journal*, 133–147.

Pennington-Zoelner, K. (2009). Expanding 'community' in the community response to intimate partner violence. *Journal of Family Violence, 24*, 539–545.

Perkins, H. W., Craig, D. W., & Perkins, J. M. (2011). Using social norms to reduce bullying: A research intervention among adolescents in five middle schools. *Group Processes & Intergroup Relations, 14*, 703–722.

PETSA. (2014). University of Montana. Accessed from http://www.umt.edu/petsa/

Polanin, J. R., Espelage, D. L., & Pigott, T. D. (2012). A meta-analysis of school-based bullying prevention programs' effects on bystander intervention behavior. *School Psychology Review, 41*, 47–65.

Potter, S. J. (2012). Using a multi-media social marketing campaign to increase active bystanders on the college campus. *Journal of American College Health, 60*, 282–295.

Potter, S. J., Moynihan, M. M., & Stapleton, J. G. (2011). Using social self-identification in social marketing materials aimed at reducing violence against women on campus. *Journal of Interpersonal Violence, 26*, 971–990.

Potter, S. J., & Stapleton, J. G. (2011). Bringing in the target audience in bystander social marketing materials for communities: Suggestions for practitioners. *Violence Against Women, 17*, 797–812.

Potter, S. J., & Stapleton, J. G. (2012). Translating sexual assault prevention from a college campus to a united states military installation: Piloting the know-your-power bystander social marketing campaign. *Journal of Interpersonal Violence, 27*, 1593–1621.

Raymond, L., Weldon, S. L., Kelly, D., Arriga, X. B., & Clark, A. M. (2014). Making change: Norm-based strategies for institutional change to address intractable problems. *Political Research Quarterly, 67*, 197–211.

RealConsent. (2014). Emory University http://emoryott.technologypublisher.com/technology/12983

Rogers, E. M. (2002). Diffusion of preventive innovations. *Addictive Behaviors, 27*, 989–993.

Roussos, S. T., & Fawcett, S. B. (2000). A review of collaborative partnerships as a strategy for improving community health. *Annual Review of Public Health, 21*, 369–402.

Ruggieria, S., Friemelb, T., Sticcac, F., Perrenc, S., & Alsaker, F. (2013). Selection and influence effects in defending a victim of bullying: The moderating effects of school context. *Procedia: Social and Behavioral Sciences, 79*, 117–126.

Sadusky, J. M., Martinson, R., Lizdas, K., & McGee, C. (2010). The praxis safety and accountability audit: Practicing a "sociology for people". *Violence Against Women, 16*(9), 1031–1044.

Mentors in Violence Prevention. http://www.mvpstrategies.net/

Red Flag Campaign. http://www.theredflagcampaign.org/

Remember Me Campaign. Accessed from http://portal.utpa.edu/utpa_main/daa_home/coah_home/pace_home/cave_home/cave_events

Safe 2 Tell. (2015). Accessed from http://safe2tell.org/

Salazar, L. F., Vivolo-Kantor, A., Hardin, J., & Berkowitz, A. (2014). A web-based sexual violence bystander intervention for male college students: Randomized control trial. *Journal of Medical Internet Research, 16*.

Sapouna, M. (2010). Collective efficacy in the school context: Does it help explain bullying and victimization among Greek primary and secondary school students? *Journal of Interpersonal Violence, 25*, 1912–1927.

Schewe, P. (2013). *Evaluation report: Agent of change, agent of change*. Retrieved at http://www.agentofchange.net/data.html

Schmid, P. C., & Schmid Mast, M. (2013). Power increases performance in a social evaluation situation as a result of decreased stress responses. *European Journal of Social Psychology, 43*, 201–211.

Schumacher, J. A., & Smith Slep, A. M. (2004). Attitudes and dating aggression: A cognitive dissonance approach. *Prevention Science, 5*, 231–243.

Scribner, R. A., Mason, K. E., Simonsen, N. R., Theall, K., Chotalia, J., Johnson, S., et al. (2010). An ecological analysis of alcohol-outlet density and campus-reported violence at 32 U.S. colleges. *Journal of Studies on Alcohol and Drugs, 71*, 184–191.

Scribner, R. A., Theall, K., Mason, K. E., Simonsen, N. R., Schneider, S. K., Towvim, L. G., & DeJong, W. (2011). Alcohol prevention on college campuses: The moderating effect of the alcohol environment on the effectiveness of social norms marketing campaigns. *Journal of Studies on Alcohol & Drugs, 72*(2), 232–239.

Seman, G. (March 9, 2015). *Where's the line? Marysville News*. Accessed from http://www.thisweeknews.com/content/stories/marysville/news/2015/03/06/wheres-the-line-campaign-bystanders-urged-to-report-instances-of-abuse.html

Sex Signals. (2014). *Catharsis production*. Accessed from http://www.catharsisproductions.com/sexsignals.php

Sherif, C. W., Kelly, M., Rodgers, H. L., Sarup, G., & Tittler, B. I. (1973). Personal involvement, social judgment, and action. *Journal of Personality and Social Psychology, 27*, 311–328.

Staggs, S. L., White, M. L., Schewe, P. A., Davis, E. B., & Dill, E. M. (2007). Changing systems by changing individuals: the incubation approach to systems change. *American Journal of Community Psychology, 39*, 365–379.

Stein, J. L. (2007). Peer educators and close friends as predictors of male college students' willingness to prevent rape. *Journal of College Student Development, 48*, 75–89.

Strang, E., & Peterson, Z. D. (2013). The relationships among perceived peer acceptance of sexual aggression, punishment certainty, and sexually aggressive behavior. *Journal of interpersonal violence, 28*, 3369–3385.

Taylor, B. G., Stein, N. D., Mumford, E. A., & Woods, D. (2013). Shifting boundaries: An experimental evaluation of a dating violence prevention program in middle schools. *Prevention Science, 14*, 64–76.

Testa, M., Hoffman, J. H., Livingston, J. A., & Turrisi, R. (2010). Preventing college women's sexual victimization through parent based intervention: A randomized control trial. *Prevention Science, 11*, 308–318.

Ullman, S. (2010). *Talking about sexual assault: Society's response to survivors*. Washington, DC: American Psychological Association.

References

van den Bos, K., Muller, P. A., & van Bussel, A. A. (2009). Helping to overcome intervention inertia in bystander's dilemmas: Behavioral disinhibition can improve the greater good. *Journal of Experimental Social Psychology, 45*, 873–878.

Velez, J. A., Manhood, C., Ewoldsen, D. R., & Moyer-Guse, E. (2012). Ingroup versus outgroup conflict in the context of violent video game play: The effect of cooperation on increasing helping and decreasing aggression. *Communication Research, 41*, 607–626.

Wandersman, A., & Florin, P. (2003). Community interventions and effective prevention. *American Psychologist, 58*, 441–448.

Wenzel, M. (2004). An analysis of norm processes in tax compliance. *Journal of Economic Psychology, 25*, 213–228.

White House Task Force to Protect Students from Sexual Assault. (2014). Notalone.gov.

White, C. H., & Malkowski, J. (2014). Communicative challenges of bystander intervention: Impact of goals and message design logic on strategies college students use to intervene in drinking situations. *Health Communication, 29*, 93–104.

Wilson, T. (2011). *Redirect: The surprising new science of psychological change*. NY: Little, Brown and Company.

White Ribbon Campaign. http://www.whiteribbon.ca/

Zimbardo, P. G., & Leippe, M. R. (1991). *The psychology of attitude change and social influence*. New York: McGraw Hill.

Zinkiewicz, L., Hammond, N., & Trapp, A. (2003). *Applying psychology disciplinary knowledge to psychology teaching and learning*. LTSN Psychology Report and Evaluation Series, 2.

Chapter 6
Prevention Springs from Action Coils: A Strategic Plan for Comprehensive Bystander-Focused Prevention

> *My friend was raped and I did not know how to go about it. I tried to I took her to [the crisis center] and my friends and I talked to her about it, but I wasn't really there for her enough.*
>
> *I wasn't equipped to handle the situation.*
>
> *[the prevention program] kind of was a starting point. And then it was kind of like. I-I kind of like figured out like..saw how much of a problem it was where I wouldn't have been aware of that before.*
>
> *I would have like talked about it sophomore and junior year too*
> —College students reflecting on bystander action related to sexual and relationship violence

Abstract This chapter outlines a strategic plan for implementing comprehensive bystander prevention efforts to address sexual and relationship abuse. The models of bystander action we have used for prevention have led us to be overly focused on intra-individual decision making and prevention strategies narrowly concentrated on one or two pieces of how and why bystanders act. A broader view considers bystanders' actions across time, both in the unfolding of the immediate risky situation, but also by considering bystander action across the lifespan. Bystander action coils also span different settings and different bystander roles. We need sets of prevention strategies for all of these time points and settings so that bystander actions spread across ecological niches. We need interventions that focus on community-level variables related to action. We need broader environments ready to have ongoing conversations with bystanders about what worked and what did not to work against entrenched stories that highlight only barriers to action. We need to consider building collective efficacy so that bystander intervention is not just about one's own actions but about how individuals can support other bystanders who step in. This chapter describes a set of ideas for next steps in this work including revising helping scripts, expanding our view of bystanders' roles, and better anticipating consequences of bystander actions.

Keywords Comprehensive prevention · Prevention settings

This chapter outlines a strategic plan for implementing comprehensive bystander prevention efforts to address sexual and relationship abuse. The models of bystander action we have used for prevention have led us to be overly focused on action coil one, intra-individual decision making. Prevention strategies have been narrowly concentrated on one or two pieces of how and why bystanders act. The broader view described in chapters four and five proposed a way of thinking about action coils across time, both in the unfolding of the immediate risky situation, but also by considering bystander action across the lifespan. Action coils also span different settings and different bystander roles. We need sets of prevention strategies for all of these settings so that bystander actions create the ripple effects needed to end violence. We need interventions that focus on community-level variables related to action. We need broader environments ready to have ongoing conversations with bystanders about their actions . We need to enhance how bystanders work together to create community-level changes (Banyard, 2013).

6.1 General Principles of Next Generation Bystander Prevention Approaches

6.1.1 Comprehensive Mobilization

The next generation of bystander prevention needs to embrace comprehensive bystander mobilization. This means teaching bystanders that helping is more than a linear process, more than a one-time intervention, and involves more than one action. The stories of several students reminds us of this, "well I've heard about it [a friend's experience of victimization] for a couple months now so like it's kind of hard to say the same things over and over and she doesn't seem to get the message but I still feel like I have to try to help her." Another student talked about the process of trying different strategies to help when their first interaction was unsuccessful. This student also described navigating potential consequences for his own safety as he walked across campus and observed what he worried was relationship violence, "well they were fighting umm it was late at night and umm he-he got very physical with her and at that point just kind of like 'hey..you know.. are you alright?' And um I was walking towards them anyways to go past and um yeah I stepped in between them and um then they started turning on me, so I just kinda, I-I walked away and called the [campus] cops and they came and took care of it…" This bystander was prepared to try several options to reduce the risk he perceived. He was prepared to read the situation as it unfolded and to stay energized while also sensitized to potential consequences.

6.1.2 Building New Helping Scripts

Preventionists should recognize that bystanders may be drawing from helping scripts that do not account for this complexity. Thus, prevention tools need to have at their center skill building exercises that help participants design and practice new things to do and say. Prevention programs should extend beyond even short term educational programs to provide bystanders with spaces to check in about their actions, seek support and advice, develop new skills and report back about negative consequences. These websites or groups could also be locations to discuss the aftermath of bystander action—whether it was well-received, whether bystanders were retaliated against, how bystanders felt about what happened. Such supportive contexts can help ensure that even if at times negative effects are experienced, these are addressed so that bystanders can build positive helping experiences that will fuel future actions. Thus prevention itself needs to be ongoing and changing to meet the needs of individuals and communities as they develop. It can not be a static program in a box.

6.1.3 Expanding View of Bystander Roles

Another component of an expanded bystander prevention model is that we need to be more intentional about naming and addressing the different roles bystanders can play. Each role carries with it a different set of potential actions. To date, bystander education seems to group behaviors together through training for general bystander action . However, it is likely that different action coils exist for each of these roles and more specific skill building may be needed for each. For example, in the supporter role with victims after an incident of SV or IPV bystanders need to have active listening skills, to know what resources are available in their community that might be useful to a survivor, and to be able to move past victim blaming attitudes they may hold so that they can give the positive disclosure reactions that promote a survivors' recovery (Ullman 2010). In the spokesperson role, however, bystanders need skills is persuasive communication as they move beyond reacting to risk or an incident to positive, protective factor building activities. For example, organizing and participating in ways of socializing that support respectful relationship, modeling media literacy about gender and sexuality, modeling ways to talk about healthy relationships, taking the lead in getting prevention and educational programs to come to organizations they are part of, mentoring young people. It is unlikely that all of these various skill sets can be taught simultaneously in one prevention program. Rather we need to see bystander intervention training as a series of prevention initiatives that over time will provide skill building across many different bystander roles. For example, bystander training could be conceptualized as a series of modules that focus on each of the five roles I described (defender, supporter, witness, spokesperson, dissenter). Following a more general foundation introduction to bystanders and why they are important, modules for each role would be layered. Each module would build skills needed for the set of behaviors that would most effectively address each role.

6.1.4 Consequences of Bystander Action

Prevention programs need to better consider consequences of bystander action and help potential bystanders think carefully about the pros and cons of what they might do. This includes explicit discussions of bystander safety as well as how the position of a bystander in the community may impact how their actions will be received. As research accumulates about what strategies are safe and that seem to work or not as bystander actions in different situations and roles, ongoing training can then help bystanders choose these more effective actions and tailor them for community-specific contexts (Potter and Stapleton 2011).

Part of considering consequences and working to make outcomes of bystander action more positive involves more fully engaging in community-wide prevention initiatives, what Wandersman and Florin (2003) describe as community-initiated and more comprehensive efforts. We need to not just change people but change contexts and remember that those contexts will vary by ecological niche. Rather than choosing a social marketing campaign or an online training why not combine them? Social marketing campaigns, messages from key community leaders, and other broad strategies can be combined with reviews of community policies for how well they support or inhibit bystander action. This also means mobilizing more than individual bystanders (usually defined as students on a campus or in a school). Below I give examples of pieces of work that could happen in different community settings. What is important is that all of these pieces need to be put in place simultaneously. The result will be broader community culture change that will both support bystanders and reduce violence. The end goal is creating communities free of IPV and SV, the best possible consequence of bystander focused prevention.

6.2 Prevention Across Levels and Settings of the Ecological Model

The following is a list of potential pieces of prevention that could be put in place in a community to better actualize the bystander action coils described in Chap. 4.

- Individuals need ongoing bystander training. This training might use narrative exercises like daily diaries to help bystanders better recognize the range of risky situations they could respond to and to build empathy for victims. These strategies can be partnered with role playing exercises and discussions to build new helping scripts and expand the individual bystander's toolkit. Social marketing

campaigns that display new norms and correct misperceptions about how often people help can be used to create new personal norms for action.
- Families are a site for modeling prosocial behavior and for reinforcing helping norms. It is also a location for ongoing discussions of what is working or not when family members try to take action. Families can support one another as engaged bystanders and parents can role model expectations about helping for children. We know prevention is more effective when parents are involved (Finkelhor et al. 2014).
- Schools are locations for workshops where skills can be developed and practiced. Classrooms can be locations for narrative "re-storying" exercises. They are also clearly marked communities where social marketing messages about norms can be displayed and more frequently seen. Faculty, staff and administrators should be part of bystander education as they are the leaders who can initiate important discussions of norms and model new behaviors. They can build collective efficacy by identifying risky hotspots and making plans for better staffing there (Taylor et al. 2013). Coaches can be enlisted as trainers of bystander messages and promoters of new peer norms (Miller et al. 2012). Prevention audits of school policies and resources can be done to make sure bystanders have safety nets to support their actions.
- Out in the community, bartenders and others can be given training as active bystanders since they are in positions to notice situations of escalating risk and since bars are another location where bystanders to sexual assault are present (BARCC: Collective Action for Safe Spaces BARCC 2014; Safe Bars 2014; Graham et al. 2014; Hensell 2014).
- Community youth and spiritual organizations can provide opportunities to practice prosocial behaviors and can be locations for ongoing discussions about bystander intervention. They are places where peer norms can be cued and developed or changed. Leaders can use cultural artifacts (including such things as passages from scripture in faith based communities or aspects of club or team identity for other organizations) that will make messages more convincing to participants and cultivate identification with new messages. Bystander action audits can be done to look at the messages organizational traditions send about helping, SV and IPV.
- Workplaces and healthcare settings have become the site of awareness campaigns and screening about SV and IPV but could also be locations for messages about bystander action.
- Government policy has already become an important part of bystander prevention with the latest amendments to the Violence Against Women Act and the White House Task Force to Protect Students From Sexual Assault (notalone. gov). College campuses are now mandated to provide some form of bystander education to college students. Faculty and staff are considered employees who are responsible for activating campus responses to SV and IPV and stalking. This is an amazing opportunity to create community change and mobilize bystanders to prevent SV and IPV. We now need to help communities make the most of this moment by helping them be creative about how to design and

resource more effective initiatives and training and encouraging research that examines their effectiveness and key active ingredients.

6.3 Promoting Bystander Action Across the Lifespan: Developmental Leverage Points

The following is a list of examples of how bystander prevention could be put in place across the lifespan (Banyard, 2013).

- Early childhood and elementary school years need to be spaces for nurturing environments (Biglan et al. 2012). Children learn perspective taking, empathy, and start building personal stories of being engaged and helpful to their family, school, and community. Bystander intervention can be a facet of moral development.
- Middle school years can focus on friendships, peer norms and skill building related to being bystanders to bullying. Parents can be trained to help cultivate positive bystander stories and to help young adolescents navigate bystander consequences and safety.
- High school students can then layer on an understanding of respectful and healthy romantic relationships with dating and sexual violence awareness and bystander training. For this age group a bystander lens might be used for a range of prevention related concerns including substance use, mental health concerns and interpersonal violence. Work on peer norms is key and it would be interesting to examine the effectiveness of Wilson's (2011) "re-storying' narratives done in peer groups to promote positive actions. These could be partnered with important community engagement activities such as the theater project described by Foshee et al. (2004). Adolescents can take active roles in creating change in their communities.
- From adolescence to young adulthood as a sense of identity continues to solidify, prevention strategies can continue to focus on developing bystander action as a focus of personal identity stories. Bystander identities across various roles can be promoted including seeing oneself not only as a supporter of a friend who is a victim, but as a proactive innovator of social justice ideas, as an early adopter of new norms and as a supporter of other bystanders. Taking advantage of key developmental transitions, campuses might start with Testa's (2010) parent intervention before students come to campus. Students could also take an online training on sexual and relationship violence and bystanders as well. As students arrive on campus eager for new friendships, they can be trained in the supporter bystander role. Capitalizing on their desire for social connection, such tools can teach them how to listen to a friend who may disclose their victimization and they can be taught where campus resources and reporting mechanisms are so that they can better help others. These early efforts can be followed by skill building and support for bystanders as defenders and potentially as witnesses

during students' second and third years. In their potential role as campus leaders in their senior year, students can be engaged in the spokesperson role as bystanders—training as mentors and popular opinion leaders who model new community norms for incoming students, norms that support victims and bystanders.
- For adults, support and training for bystanders can continue in communities at large via faith based communities, public service announcements, and media spotlights on the positive impact bystanders can have. Emphasis for adults can be how they can help young people become the next generation of better bystanders as well as how they can take action themselves to help coworkers and neighbors. Training in workplace or neighborhood groups can focus on increasing collective efficacy to end violence.

6.4 Conclusion

Bystander intervention is a potentially powerful prevention tool for SV and IPV that can be at the center of strategies across the social ecological model and across the lifespan. Hamby and Grych (2013) encourage us to think about how bystanders are also key linkages between forms of violence as a common protective factor. Actualizing the potential of this framework, however, requires first looking more carefully at our models for how and under what conditions safe bystander action happens and with what effects. It then requires embracing and strategically planning for a more comprehensive prevention agenda. New research is a key piece of this approach. We need to better understand what components of bystander prevention are the most active ingredients and what combination of strategies have the biggest impact while conserving resources. This work can lead not only to better bystanders but to community wide action coils that move us toward ending not just sexual and relationship violence but many forms of victimization.

References

Banyard, V. L. (2013). Go big or go home: Reaching for a more integrated view of violence prevention. (Peer reviewed commentary). *Psychology of Violence, 3*, 115–120.
BARCC. (2014). *Boston Area Rape Crisis Center*. http://www.barcc.org/active/bars
Biglan, A., Flay, B. R., Embry, D. D., & Sandler, I. N. (2012). The critical role of nurturing environments for promoting human well-being. *American Psychologist, 67*, 257–271.
Finkelor, D., Vanderminden, J., Turner, H., Shattuck, A., & Hamby, S. (2014). Youth exposure to violence prevention programs in a national sample. *Child Abuse and Neglect, 38*, 677–686.
Foshee, V. A., Bauman, K. E., Ennett, S. T., Linder, G. F., Benefield, T., & Suchindran, C. (2004). Assessing the long-term effects of the safe dates program and a booster in preventing and reducing adolescent dating violence victimization and perpetration. *American Journal of Public Health, 94*, 619–624.
Graham, K., Bernards, S., Osgood, D. W., Abbey, A., Parks, M., Flynn, A., et al. (2014). "Blurred lines?" Sexual aggression and barroom culture. *Alcoholism, Clinical and Experimental Research, 38*, 1416–1424.

Hamby, S., & Grych, J. (2013). *The web of violence: Exploring connections among different forms of interpersonal violence and abuse*. Dordrecht, Netherlands: Springer.

Hensell, C. (2014). *Arizona's Bar Bystander Project*. Accessed from http://www.azrapeprevention.org/sites/azrapeprevention.org/files/adhs_may_update.pdf

Miller, E., Tancredi, D. J., McCauley, H. L., Decker, M. R., Virata, M. C., Anderson, H. A., Stetkevich, N., Brown, E. W., Miodeen, F., & Silverman, J. (2012). "Coaching boys into men": A cluster-randomized controlled trial of a dating violence prevention program. *Journal of Adolescent Health, 51*, 431–438.

Potter, S. J., & Stapleton, J. G. (2011). Bringing in the target audience in bystander social marketing materials for communities: Suggestions for practitioners. *Violence Against Women, 17*, 797–812.

Safe Bars. (2014). Accessed from http://www.collectiveactiondc.org/programs/safe-bars/

Taylor, B. G., Stein, N D., Mumford, E. A., & Woods, D. (2013). Shifting boundaries: An experimental evaluation of a dating violence prevention program in middle schools. *Prevention Science, 14*, 64–76.

Testa, M., Hoffman, J. H., Livingston, J. A., & Turrisi, R. (2010). Preventing college women's sexual victimization through parent based intervention: A randomized control trial. *Prevention Science, 11*, 308–318.

Ullman, S. (2010). *Talking about sexual assault: Society's response to survivors*. Washington, DC: American Psychological Association.

Wandersman, A., & Florin, P. (2003). Community interventions and effective prevention. *American Psychologist, 58*, 441–448.

Wilson, T. (2011). *Redirect: The surprising new science of psychological change*. NY: Little, Brown and Company.

CPI Antony Rowe
Eastbourne, UK
November 17, 2019